HEAL THYSELF!

Massage works . . . but how does it work? And what does it do? It can speed up the circulation of the blood, it can help lymph circulation, it can affect muscles throughout the body, it can increase the body's secretions and excretions. It can affect the nervous system, it can soothe you—not only physically, but psychologically. It can enhance skin luster and beauty. Western therapies utilize massage for headache, for cough or hoarseness, for hiccoughs, for smarting or burning eyes, even for toothache, massage can help.

This new, complete guide to sensual health through massage will show you how.

MASSAGE:
The Touching Way to Sensual Health

Massage:
The Touching Way To Sensual Health

BY CONSTANCE YOUNG

Illustrated by Sandy Kossin

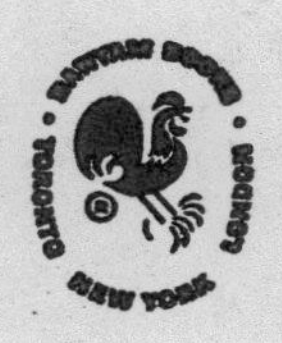

MASSAGE: THE TOUCHING WAY TO SENSUAL HEALTH
A Bantam Book / June 1975

Published simultaneously in the United States and Canada

Bantam Books are published by Bantam Books, Inc. Its trademark, consisting of the words "Bantam Books" and the portrayal of a bantam, is registered in the United States Patent Office and in other countries. Marca Registrada. Bantam Books, Inc., 666 Fifth Avenue, New York, New York 10019.

PRINTED IN THE UNITED STATES OF AMERICA

I believe a leaf of grass is no less than the
journey-work of the stars,
And the pismire is equally perfect, and a grain of
sand, and the egg of the wren,
And the tree-toad is a chef-d'oeuvre for the highest,
And the running blackberry would adorn the parlors of
heaven,
And the narrowest hinge in my hand puts to scorn
all machinery . . .

—*Walt Whitman,* Song of Myself

Contents

4

The Basic "How-To's" 35

Introduction

This book is about energy.

It is about the energy exchanged between two people during the communication of massage. But more important, it is about energy coursing through the body as a person receives a massage.

There are many names for this formerly intangible thing—orgone energy, chi, ki, impulses, bioplasma, aura, electron emission, corona discharge and life fields. It has long been sensed, but it can now presumably be seen and photographed using a technique called Kirlian photography.*

This "life force" or "spark of life" *does* exist, and it does change, and in this book I show how to move it about and use it to one's best advantage through massage.

---

* Kirlian photography was discovered by a Russian electrician in 1939. It is a means of photographing objects using high voltage spark discharges and *no* camera or lens. A generator is used to create the electrical field, and it is attached to a plate, some photosensitive paper, and the subject.

1

Massage Works . . . And How

Man is born whole and can remain whole,
but usually lives in a state of disharmony.
*—Gertrude Enelow**

It's not a cure-all, but massage can heal; it's a fact! How it works is not thoroughly understood. And there is still controversy surrounding it. For one thing, there are those who practice massage who are not reliable or capable. The shady "massage parlors" haven't helped the image of the reputable masseurs. But, fortunately, in spite of this, massage is generally accepted in orthodox medical circles, and drugless medical techniques are coming more and more into their own. The incursions of Chinese medical systems, such as acupuncture, into the practice of Western medicine have a great deal to do with it. There is also a growing acceptance of "body-mind unity," and all illnesses—both the somatic and the psychic—are less likely to be thought of as emanating from either the body alone or the mind alone. Plainly what this means in terms of our everyday experience is that the athlete might do well to practice yoga or meditation to help relieve his "kinks," or an intellectual, when blocked from doing a mental task by a headache, might do well to have a massage to get his head "working" again. The body is less likely to be thought of as a kind of second cousin

* from *Body Dynamics*, New York Citadel Press, 1963

to the mind or "spirit" as it once was. The days are gone, fortunately, when people thought like the American poet Frederick Lawrence Knowles, who, in the late 1800's wrote, "The body is my house—it is not I: Triumphant in this faith I live and die." But rather, most of us realize that we are our bodies. As Swineburne wrote, "Body and spirit are twins. . . ."

There are believers and nonbelievers, but even a diehard nonbeliever has to agree that massage has some effect on the body, and all of its good results cannot just be attributed to "faith healing" or the "placebo effect." Recent innovations in electronics have also contributed to this growing acceptance of massage. For one thing, changes in the body can be clearly seen with the latest electronic equipment. In one study done at a major medical center in this country*, the following occurred after a conventional back massage: blood pressure, increased; heart rate, increased; sweat-gland activity, increased; peripheral skin temperature, increased; general body temperature, increased; pupil diameter, increased; and respiration rate, decreased.

All the preceding were the tests used to show the state of a person's autonomic nervous system. The study concluded ". . . that massage does have an influence on the autonomic functions of the body."

Even the prestigious American Medical Association, in a recent handbook, reported that oxygen consumption goes up from ten to fifteen percent after either a general massage or an abdominal massage.

Although it is still uncertain exactly what happens in the body after massage, some generalizations can be made.

---

* The study was performed by J. S. Barr and N. Taslitz. Mrs. Barr is an Associate in Physical Therapy at Duke University Medical Center and Dr. Taslitz is Assistant Professor of Physical Therapy and Professor of Anatomy at Case Western Reserve University.

What Happens Physiologically

The use of massage cuts across many disciplines. It is used by M.D.s, osteopaths, acupuncturists, physical therapists, yogis, psychologists, psychiatrists, masseurs or masseuses, dancers, naturapaths, members of the Human Potential movement, sex therapists, and so on. For this book I have tried to reach some consensus among these different theories. The yogi might talk about "prana," the Reichian psychologist might speak of "orgone" energy, the M.D. might simply speak of the neural reflexes; but by whatever name it is called, some intangible energy is manipulated and changed in some way through massage. All will also agree that massage improves the circulation of the blood. And anyone who's had a general massage by a good and reputable practitioner will join in the unanimous opinion that "massage feels good." I can vouch for it myself; I've had many a massage, and it does certainly make you feel good.

Leaving aside the Oriental theory of medicine, which is discussed in a later chapter and which embodies totally unique doctrines not generally understood by those accustomed to Western medicine, massage is known to:

1. *Speed up the circulation of the blood.* According to Beard's textbook of massage* for physical therapists, there are several studies, in addition to the Barr-Taslitz study previously mentioned, which prove increases in blood circulation following massage. In some of these studies, small superficial blood vessels (called capillaries) that are not visible under normal circumstances

* Beard, G., and Wood, E. E.: *Massage, Principles and Techniques*, Philadelphia and London, W. B. Saunders Company, 1964.

are clearly seen after a person is massaged. This is attributable to increased volume of blood surging through them.

This increase of circulation is thought to occur from either of two effects. The first is the *mechanical* effect. This means that massage works something like squeezing a tube of toothpaste. When the muscles of the body are relaxed, the fluid (blood) within the tubes (blood vessels) is pushed in the direction in which the pressure is applied. Massage is usually conducted toward the center of the body or the heart (or in the direction of the veins, which send blood to the heart). It would follow that since the amount of blood brought through the veins to the heart is increased by massage, the rate of heartbeat should be increased, and thus a greater amount of arterial blood should be carried away from the heart toward the body. The arteries lie deeper in the body, so they are less likely to be affected by direct mechanical stimulation.

In the other effect of massage, or the "reflex" effect, the nervous system comes into play. When the skin is lightly massaged, receptors there are stimulated. This transmits signals to the brain, which causes the blood vessels to dilate.

2. *Cause changes in the blood.* There is an increase in the oxygen capacity of the blood after massage. A few early studies show an increase in the red blood count and in the hemoglobin (the oxygen-carrying red pigment of the red blood corpuscles) after either a general or abdominal massage. In another study, after a local massage, there was an increase in the platelet count in that area. (Platelets are cells found in the blood which help it to clot. Without enough platelets in the blood a person might hemorrhage when cut.)

3. *Help lymph circulation.* Lymph is a fluid containing a type of white blood cell, called lymphocytes, and

moving through channels not unlike blood vessels. Spaced throughout this lymphatic system are glandlike structures, or nodes, which act as valves. The major function of the lymph is to fight infection, and it tends to gather where there is an area of disease or trauma. But lymph sometimes strays from the vessels and invades the surrounding areas, because lymph does not circulate as the blood does, aided by a pumping heart. The movement of lymph depends largely on external factors, such as massage. This is why massage is particularly useful in conditions such as arthritis, in which lymph tends to remain stagnant in the affected areas, thereby increasing a person's discomfort. In addition, when lymph strays, massage helps to coax it back into the vessels.

4. *Affect muscles throughout the body.* There have been a number of studies concerned with the effect of massage on the muscles. Most agree that it cannot increase muscle strength. But it can promote recovery from fatigue that occurs after excessive exercise. In this way it can make it possible to do more exercise, which may in the long run strengthen the muscles. Massage also helps heal injured muscles. And perhaps the greatest benefit of massage is its ability to keep the muscles in the best possible state of nutrition, pliancy, and vitality.

5. *Increase the body's secretions and excretions.* There is a proven increase in urination following massage—particularly abdominal massage—which can last for several days. In addition to helping rid the body of poisons and waste products of fatigue, another advantage of this increased output of urine is a loss of weight, albeit temporary. There are also some masseurs who claim that local massage can remove fat deposits from

various regions of the body, but this has not been proven. I have seen in myself what looked like a loss of fat around my middle after massage. But this was, in fact, a redistribution of weight through a stretching out of my body, which can occur after more exotic methods such as Alexander technique and rolfing, both of which I explain in detail later.

That massage has some effect on the metabolism was proven some fifty years ago, when, as mentioned in Beard's textbook, it was discovered that there was an increase in the rate of excretion of nitrogen, inorganic phosphorus, and sodium chloride (salt) after massage. These chemicals are all byproducts of metabolism.

Studies indicate that fluids surrounding the tissues being massaged are dispersed. There are also some claims of improved general cell nutrition.

6. *Affect the nervous system.* It has been observed for some years that certain kinds of pain can be relieved by massage. How this is accomplished is not certain. When we consider the pronounced sedative effect massage produces—one masseuse I interviewed considers it flattery to her skill when one of her clients falls asleep while being massaged—there has to be some effect on the central nervous system. Peripheral nerves are also soothed by gentle stroking; one can actually feel the nerve endings tingle.

7. *Have a psychological effect.* Due to the practitioner's concentrated attention on the subject, combined with the pleasant sensations massage can induce, there is often a close relationship brought about that causes the person being massaged to reveal things he usually keeps secret. When a person is ill, just the knowledge that something is being done may relieve some of his anxiety about his illness.

8. *Enhance skin luster and beauty.* Because the capillaries expand, there is increased nourishment to the body's glands and superficial tissues. The nervous system is also stimulated. All this improves the general appearance. The complexion and texture of the skin are healthier and the color is better due to the increased circulation and increased body temperature. Psychologically, it is also true that if we feel better, we look better.

Some Specific Contributions and Cures

Massage has been used to stimulate or restore various internal organs. The most dramatic and successful use of massage for an internal organ is on the heart, in the so-called cardiac massage. In 1960 Dr. Kouwenhoven and his associates* reported a seventy-percent survival rate for those patients with a cardiac arrest who received massage. For best results, as in all cases where internal organs are involved, it should be done by an expert. But during the time you're waiting for a doctor to arrive when a person's heart has stopped, it would be well to know what to do; that's why in Chapter VI we demonstrate this life-saving cardiac-massage technique.

Abdominal massage is another treatment that is often used to increase peristaltic action and thus remove wastes and gases from the intestines. This is good particularly in very old people and in those who are bedridden.

Another organ which responds to massage is the gallbladder. And for years doctors were performing the difficult prostatic massage on patients with an obstructed prostate. This was performed directly on the prostate

---

* Beard, *op. cit.*

gland, with instruments. They've since stopped doing it because the instruments may induce infection. But these are all considerations for a physician, as massage of this nature should never be done by a layperson.

In dentistry, too, massage has its uses. This is particularly so as a daily measure for the prevention of gum disorders.

Aside from its use outside medicine for general relaxation and improvement in circulation, massage is used in orthodox medicine for a wide variety of diseases or trauma of the muscles and joints; these include rheumatism, arthritis, sprains and strains, tired feet, leg cramps, backache, and so forth. In Oriental medicine it is recommended for an even wider range of disorders, including diabetes, bedwetting, and deafness.

2

From Huang Ti To Esalen And Beyond

Sensory experience is not an unreliable step to knowledge, but is actually man's very gateway to the world.
*—Erwin Straus, M.D.**

Like most art, literature, and medicine, massage probably developed out of experience in the days before recorded history. People touched each other and it felt good. They rubbed herbs and oils on their bodies and noticed improvement in their ailing muscles and joints and observed that comfort and healing were achieved. One handbook used in medical schools claims that massage may be the oldest of all remedies, because it is instinctive in man as well as lower animals. Have you ever noticed a cat rub his neck and back against a surface?

The oldest written records of principles of healing were written on "oracle bones," and the earliest transcribed manuscript which mentions massage was the classical Chinese text which is the basis of the Chinese system of medicine. Called *The Yellow Emperor's Classic of Internal Medicine*, the *Huang Ti Nei Ching Su Wen*, this classic text was attributed by some to Huang Ti, the so-called Yellow Emperor, who was said to have ruled about 2697–2597 B.C. Others feel that it is unlikely that the Yellow Emperor was the actual

* from The Primary World of Senses. A Vindication of Sensory Experience, Straus, 1963

author, claiming the book was written anywhere between that time and 1000 B.C. Whatever the true authorship, it is still the oldest medical book extant. And it presents a vivid theory of medicine, much as the physicians of India provided in their classical books of medicine, or the codes of the Hippocratic physicians of Greece.

Recently translated into English, *The Yellow Emperor's Classic of Internal Medicine* deals with ancient ideas which can still be applied today, such as in the conversation between Ch'i Po and the emperor in which the emperor asks if there is any reason to supplement the treatment of acupuncture when a procedure called "draining" is done. Ch'i Po answers that "one must first feel with the hand and trace the system of the body. One should interrupt the sufficiencies and distribute them evenly, one should apply binding and massage." Later it is mentioned that when the "... body is frequently startled and frightened, the circulation in the arteries and the veins ceases, and disease arises from numbness and lack of sensation. In order to cure this, one uses massage and medicines prepared from the lees of wine (the remnants of the fermentation process)." So massage was evidently used when there were apparent difficulties of circulation.

Independently, systems of massage developed among the ancient Hindus, Persians, and Egyptians. When Alexander invaded India he found that the king liked to be massaged while he received visitors. Elegant ladies at the time of Cleopatra were massaged by servants as they bathed in gallons of perfumed water. This, of course, was as much for beauty and pleasure as for therapy. There has always been a close relationship between the sensuous and the therapeutic elements in massage.

But it was the Greeks who appeared to refine the technique of massage for use by the Western world, and they used it for healing as well as relief of pain. The word "massage" comes from the Greek word *massein*, "to knead," although even the Greeks knew that massage meant more than a mere kneading of muscle. As far back as the Homeric Age (1000 B.C.) the Greeks recognized the restorative value of anointing one's body with oils. Homer describes Odysseus' homecoming, when he was bathed and "anointed . . . with olive oil, and . . . he came forth from the bath in fashion like the deathless gods." Herodikus (circa 500 B.C.) and Herodotus (484–424 B.C.) also described the use of massage. The great Plato, in the late fifth and early fourth century B.C., received regular massage until he died at the age of more than one hundred. Hippocrates, who lived about 460–377 B.C. and is called the "Father of (modern) Medicine," described massage as part of his total treatment program. In the case of constipation, he advocated kneading. In general, he wrote that "hard rubbing binds; soft rubbing loosens; much rubbing causes parts to waste; moderate rubbing makes them grow." The great medical authority Galen (A.D. 130–200) developed a complete procedure and technique for therapeutic massage.

The Romans knew of massage too, for Asclepiades, a fashionable Roman physician, who was a Greek by birth, declared that massage was an important aid toward building a healthy and attractive body. Cicero and Pliny, not to mention the great Caesar himself, were advocates of regular massage. After a great surge of popularity among the great philosophers, physicians, and rulers, it gradually faded in popularity.

Meanwhile, in China, its use continued. There appears to be a direct relationship between pressure on various skin points (acupuncture points) and the health of internal organs. Massage of these points is used to relieve many illnesses just as needles are also used to cure or relieve disease. As massage techniques developed gradually along with acupuncture, every little town in China had a practitioner trained to do acupuncture and/or massage, each with his own "style." In the Western world, massage's popularity waned through most of the sixteenth and seventeenth centuries except among the few rich and pampered who could afford care. There were the few dramatic instances such as when Mary, Queen of Scots, in 1566 protracted typhus and might have died had it not been for vigorous massage. During this period fads came and went; there were the "flagellations" and "magnetic" touches which took the place of serious therapeutic development. It might be called the "Dark Age" of massage. One bright note: in France in the eighteenth century Voltaire popularized the so-called *trémoussoire*, the forerunner of today's vibrating chair.

In the beginning of the nineteenth century a Swedish fencing master, Peter Henrik Ling, introduced a system of movement that consisted of massage and exercises. This regimen synthesized the then-existing European massage practices with those used in the Orient. This method spread throughout Europe and became the basis for what is now known as Swedish massage. Later the Frenchman Just Lucas-Championnière introduced a more gentle type of massage in which strokes were slow, uniform, rhythmic, and "little more than a caress." James B. Mennell of England borrowed from Lucas-Championnière and systematized the massage movements even further so that they applied to the treatment of many more conditions. His work has had a great influence on today's use of massage in the practice of medicine in the United States and England.

This is essentially how massage came to be used as an adjunct to the practice of medicine. In other spheres, particularly the psychophysical, the development took a slightly different turn.

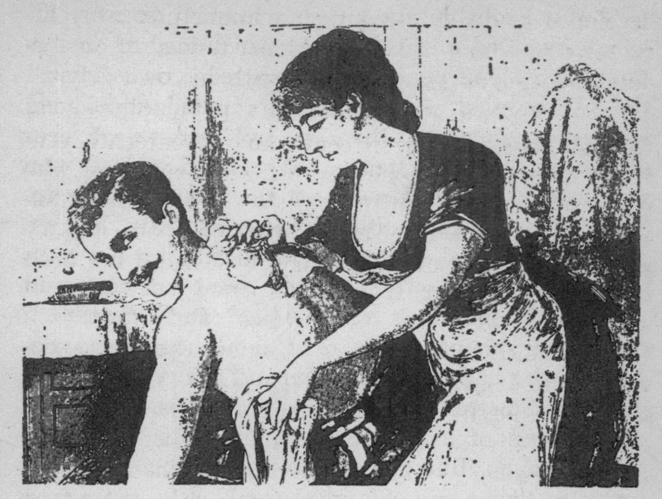

Rubbing Hubby's back. Woodcut, 1884. *(Courtesy The Bettman Archive, New York.)*

To understand the development of massage techniques as they are now used in healing on a more psychological level, we must look at history somewhat differently. Let us start with the "Nature Cure." Its basic theory was, and still is, that if the body is nourished only with the ingredients that it needs, and if ingredients that are harmful are excluded, the body will avoid disease; or if disease strikes, it will be able to throw illness off by its own unaided efforts, without recourse to drugs or surgery. The foundation stone of this Nature Cure was what Hippocrates defined as *vis medicatrix naturae*, or the body's recuperative powers, the "life force." This became the essential premise of naturopathic medicine, and part of the nature "cure" consisted of massage. During ancient times physicians of the Aesculapian order had established temples of health where patients were put through a course of bathing and massage. These Aesculapian temples were probably not unlike a faddish British resort which bloomed in the 1940s to which the rich and famous went. This popular establishment was a cross between a hospital and a luxury hotel; the affluent and upwardly mobile went there and lived for two weeks on orange juice and raw salad, and received hydrotherapy and osteopathic treatment, and of course massage. Such hotels still exist, although on a smaller scale.

Osteopathy had developed out of another old medical system—bone-setting. Since humans started to walk on two legs, they have always been susceptible to strains and sprains, and in time, there came to be individuals who had a knack of putting things right again. These bonesetters were considered by the M.D.s as practitioners of a vulgar knack that was little more than a hobby. But out of this finally emerged osteopathic medicine and chiropractic, which form the basis for some of the body-mind healing techniques that utilize massage.

Then in the late 1800s and early 1900s came Freud and psychoanalysis. A young psychiatrist and colleague of Freud's, Sândor Ferenczi, accepted Freud's basic assumptions but made changes and modifications that brought him into frequent conflict with Freud. His major innovation was the introduction of "activity techniques." These took many forms: In 1923 he reported on the use of relaxation exercises to help his patients in their treatment and also reported on their muscular activity during these exercises.

In 1942, another renegade went further to describe what he called "muscular armor." Wilhelm Reich felt that it was possible to determine the character type of a person either by a study of his behavior or by an analysis of his bodily attitudes. The concept was that, like a medieval knight, a person built a muscular armor as his defense, and like all armor, the character armor creates a limitation in body movement and decreases a person's sensitivity. In Australia F. Matthias Alexander also developed an approach to body-mind using a light form of touching—work which was to greatly influence many famous people, including George Bernard Shaw, John Dewey, and Aldous Huxley. Then at Esalen in Big Sur, California, there was a renaissance of the psychotherapies, and some new and dramatic forms grew and matured. Most—like the dramatic and radical body work by Ida Rolf, called structural integration—rely heavily on the "muscular-armor" concept of Wilhelm Reich. Ida Rolf's type of massage work attempts to physically rebuild a "new person" freed of destructive bodily attitudes and centered in gravity. She systematically molds the subject's connective tissue, which surrounds every one of the major muscle systems, much as one would mold a piece of clay.

Fritz Perls, a Gestalt therapist, in describing his personal goals, speaks for most of this human potential movement. The key word for all of them is true development of the "whole" person, and the goals are ". . . to become real, to learn to take a stand, to develop one's center. . . ." Those goals may be reached through the body and/or the mind, and one of their tools is massage—but systematically applied, in a very different way.

Where once there was only Esalen at Big Sur, groups with similar goals have sprouted up all over the country. There is now Aureon Institute, Anthos, and the National Institute for the Psychotherapies in New York City; Tarrytown House in Tarrytown, New York, to name only a few on the East Coast. Many large universities and colleges throughout the country now have courses in "human potential." (For the name of a group in your area, write to Esalen at Big Sur or any of the above and tell them of your primary interest.)

Another new area of massage has grown out of the sex research of Masters and Johnson; the ancient practice of erotic massage is becoming formularized for people needing treatment for sexual problems. To my mind this shows an encouraging new acceptance of touch as a mode of communication, for part of what makes a good massage makes a good sexual relationship—that is, experimentation and an open give-and-take of sensual pleasure.

Two additional massage techniques, zone therapy and polarity therapy, have relatively few followers.

The purpose of this book is to gather the best of the old and the new systems and compile them into a practical survey. What can be taught in a book of this kind is given with easy-to-follow instructions and illustrations. Those techniques that require greater skill and training are described so that the reader can know what they are and where to find a reliable or authorized practitioner.

3

The Basic Massage Strokes

Every man is the builder of a temple,
called his body.

—*Thoreau*

There are several basic movements at the root of all systems of massage the names may vary from system to system, but the principles remain the same. Some movements are applicable to all parts of the body, others only to specific areas. Where a particular stroke is contraindicated in an area, I am careful to mention it. Usually, however, if the wrong stroke is used, the person doing the massage soon becomes well aware of it by the displeased response from the subject. For the most part, there is room for trial and error once certain important massage rules are followed. These basic rules are given at the end of this chapter.

As mentioned earlier, experimentation is an important aspect of recent developments in massage, and this is obvious by the names of some of the new strokes: "rocking horse," "swimming," "raking," where once only such names as "kneading" and "petrissage" were used. One physical therapist I interviewed mentioned that he wasn't sure of the names of the strokes he used; his technique, as that of all people doing massage, developed largely out of trial and error, as in any other "art form." The human potential movement may use the new "rocking horse" or "swimming," but it still uses age-old techniques—Chinese "cupping," for one, which dates back at least 2,500 years. I include some of the old and much of the new, in order to present the best of all methods.

All massage movements fall basically into three categories: stroking, (also called effleurage), compression, and percussion (also called tapotement). Every person doing massage has his or her own method of using these movements. They can be varied by pressure, direction, or the part of the hand being used. One masseur may use one hand for a stroke; one may use both hands. But the massage should always be performed at a uniform rate of speed and in a slow and even rhythm. At almost all times throughout the massage, one hand is always kept in contact with the subject's body.

Stroking

In the Bible and in Homer's *Odyssey* when they speak of "anointing thyself with oil," they were very likely referring to the stroking movement. To my knowledge it is used in all systems of massage.

Generally, stroking, or effleurage, is of two types—superficial or deep. The term effleurage is usually used in Western massage when referring to a light pressure, and this includes strokes with the fingertips alone as well as return strokes with the whole hand.

The usual procedure for stroking is to hold hands palms down, fingers close together and cupped to fit the contours of the subject's body. The thumbs may be spread or closed. One or both hands are used, depending on the area of the body or on the practitioner's preference.

The direction of the stroke—particularly in deep stroking—should be centripetal, or toward the center. This means that most deep stroking is done in the direction of the heart or in the direction of the veins that bring blood to the heart. Stroking is also done following the contours of a muscle. It is sometimes helpful to study a chart of the main muscle groups of the body before doing a massage for the first time. But even without such a chart, if the person doing the massage is really attuned to the other person's body as well as to his own, and if the massage is conducted gently at first, with pressure built up as needed, the muscles can be felt under the fingers. It is a little more difficult to do this during superficial stroking, as there is rarely enough pressure applied to define the muscles with the fingers.

It is important to maintain a uniform and unvarying pressure during each stroke, and when moving from stroke to stroke and area to area, and always to keep one hand lightly in contact with the subject's body. There may be times when contact must be lost briefly, but this will seldom happen during a movement. If, at the end of a stroke, hands must briefly lose contact, a rhythmic and gentle motion should be maintained so that the moment of noncontact acts something like a pause in music. Any abruptness of movement might jolt the person being massaged out of his or her relaxed mood.

Superficial stroking requires the use of extremely light pressure, much as Lucas-Championnière described—"little more than a caress." Usually the entire hand is used, with fingers held together and the thumb spread or opened to suit the needs of the part of the body being massaged. In superficial stroking, movements may be centrifugal, or away from the heart. This is true for legs and arms, because the hair falls that way and the usual centripetal strokes might be uncomfortable.

The Oriental method of stroking is similar to the Western method. The rubbing and stroking are usually done with the hand flat on the body or with the balls of the fingers alone. In Japan there is also a complete system of fingertip massage, called *Shiatsu,* in which specific points on the body (acupuncture points) are pressed.

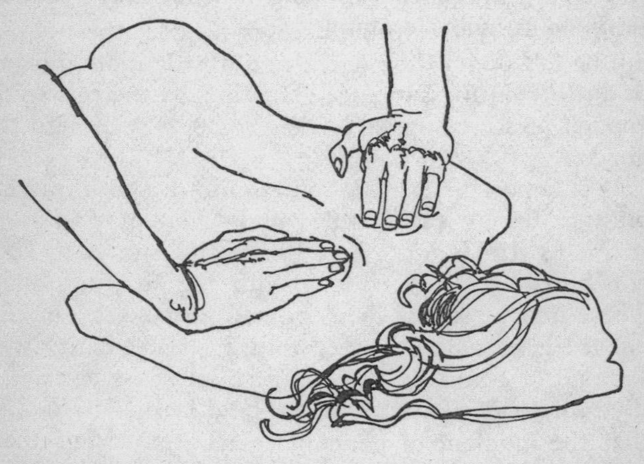

Deep stroking is done with sufficient pressure to produce mechanical effects as well as reflex effects; the blood is actually squeezed and pushed through the veins so that it flows more rapidly to the heart. In deep stroking, movements are *always* performed in the direction of the veins, or toward the heart. The purpose of this deep-stroking massage is generally to assist the venous and lymphatic circulation. Such stroking relieves fatigue and improves the tone of the skin and muscles. To perform deep massage, any part of one hand or both hands could be used. Usually it's done with the entire hand. The hand is kept in contact with the body during the entire stroke to avoid stimulating the nervous system by breaking contact with the skin. During return strokes, pressure is kept light, as in superficial stroking, so that it does not interfere with the mechanical effect of the deep stroke. Deep stroking should not induce pain under ordinary circumstances. Pressure should be uniform and vary only according to the bulk of the massage being massaged or the body type being manipulated. (A frail girl will usually require less pressure than a bulky, muscular male.)

Usually, superficial stroking is done prior to deep stroking to help the muscles relax.

Compression

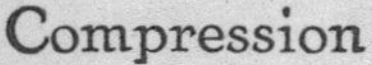

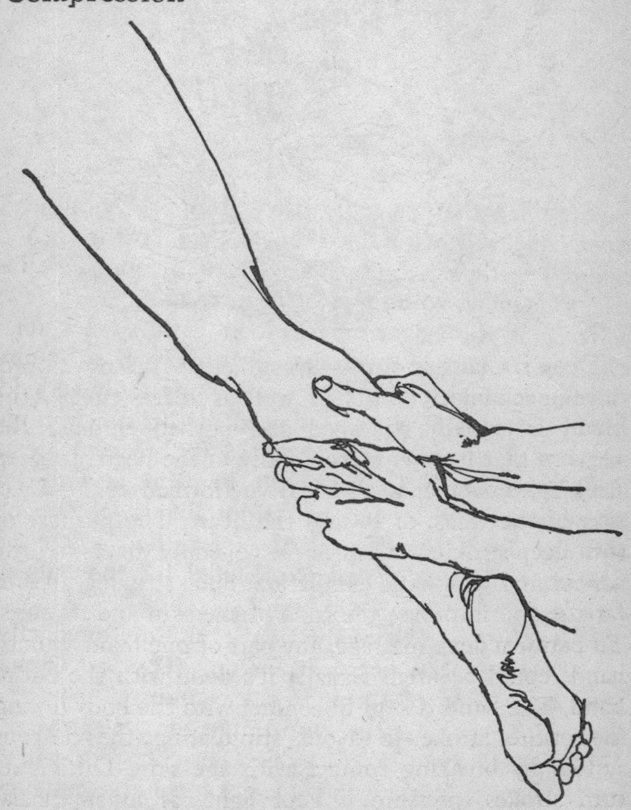

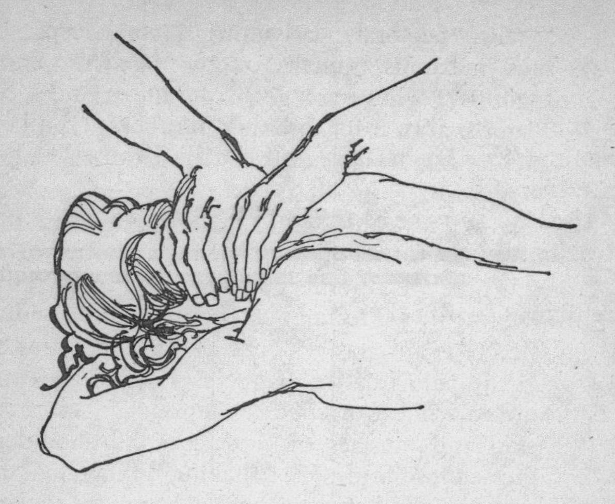

Kneading. Some people use the term "kneading," interchangeably with the French word "petrissage." I call it kneading because it's easier and more descriptive. Generally, kneading is very relaxing.

To do it, the masseur grasps loose flesh . . . or a muscle . . . or a part of a muscle . . . between the thumbs and fingers, taking as much as can comfortably be held onto. The muscle is then allowed to slip slowly from between the fingers. It is repeated for adjacent areas. Kneading may also be done with the palms or with the thumbs and the second and third fingers of one or both hands—whatever works best for the masseur or subject. Usually both hands are used for the bulkier muscles.

Movements are kept slow, gentle, and rhythmic, and care must be taken to avoid pinching. The part of the hand being used conforms to the contour of the area, As a rule, heavy pressure is directed toward the veins and heart. The muscles for which kneading works best are the larger, thicker ones of the torso and extremities, or those which are usually extremely tight or tense (trapezius, pectorals, latissimus dorsi, triceps, biceps gluteus maximus, gracilis, rectus femorus, and gastrocnemius). These are generally the muscles of the neck, upper arms, back, hips and buttocks.

Oriental kneading massage. The ancient Chinese system contains many shaking or vibrating movements that are at first gentle and then gradually build up in intensity. They are used to tone up the muscles and joints. There are a number of variations of the grasping movement: (1) "rolling of the muscles": individual muscle cords are grasped between the fingertips or between the palms of the hands and rolled backward or forward in a linear or circular motion; (2) "shrinking": the skin and muscles of the neck and shoulders are compressed into folds; (3) "shaking": individual muscle cords are grasped between the fingertips and shaken vigorously backward and forward. This is done for the arms, legs, neck, and back.

In modern Japanese systems, which are based on the ancient Chinese, kneading is done either with the thumb and index finger or with all four fingers, or the middle finger alone. The tendons which cross the joints are massaged in this manner. This motion is supposed to break up any pathological deposits that may collect in these areas, and relieve symptoms that occur after an acute attack of rheumatism of the joints has subsided. It is thought to correct the enlargement and hardening that make the joints difficult to bend, as well as bring relief to some cases of partial paralysis.

Friction. Physical therapists consider these movements good for loosening scars and helping to absorb fluids around joints. The whole palm can be used, or part of the palm, or the thumb or fingers alone. These strokes are done by moving the superficial tissues over the underlying structures by keeping the hand in firm contact and making circular movements over a small area at a time. Pressure should be firm but not heavy. The part of the hand being used is always in contact with the subject's skin.

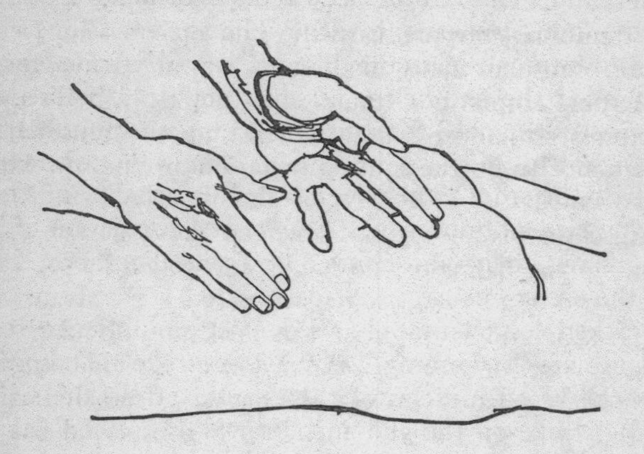

Percussion

There are any number of percussion movements that date back to ancient Rome, when masseurs used a wooden palette to restore tone to the body. The movements are usually brief, brisk, and rapidly applied contacts with one hand or both hands alternately. There is "hacking"—done with the outer border of the hand, or the relaxed fingers, bouncing the hands alternately off the part being treated as in the drawing above. It may also be done with a kind of whipping motion, using fingers as the flexible portion of the whip. There is also "clapping," in which the fingers and palms form a concave surface. If the hands are cupped, there is a deeper sound. "Beating" is done with the fists half-closed or closed. Then, also, there is "tapping," which is done with the tips of the fingers. None of the movements are intended to produce pain, but to stimulate the body.

Vibration and shaking movements are sometimes included among the percussive movements. Vibration is produced by placing the fingertips in contact with the skin, and shaking the entire arm, thereby transmitting a trembling movement to the subject.

Professional masseurs like to do percussive movements at the end of the session. But Beard's textbook expresses the need for caution and urges physical therapists not to do these movements on any person with a serious disorder. They feel that the benefits of these percussive motions, which is increased circulation of the capillaries, may be achieved by other methods, such as the use of heat.

Other, less commonly used Western massage techniques are "swimming," which is a stroke that is good for the broad muscles of the thorax. To do the swimming stroke on the abdomen, hands are placed flat on either side, with fingers pointing toward each other to the center. Hands should glide, pressing gently to the opposite side. This should be a gradual movement up and down the abdomen and chest. Then there are such strokes as "throwing," "shaking," "pulling," and "sawing," which are essentially what their names imply. To "throw" the subjects arm, do just that; "shaking" a limb or "pulling," also need no explanation.

Sawing is often done on the waistline as shown the drawing below.

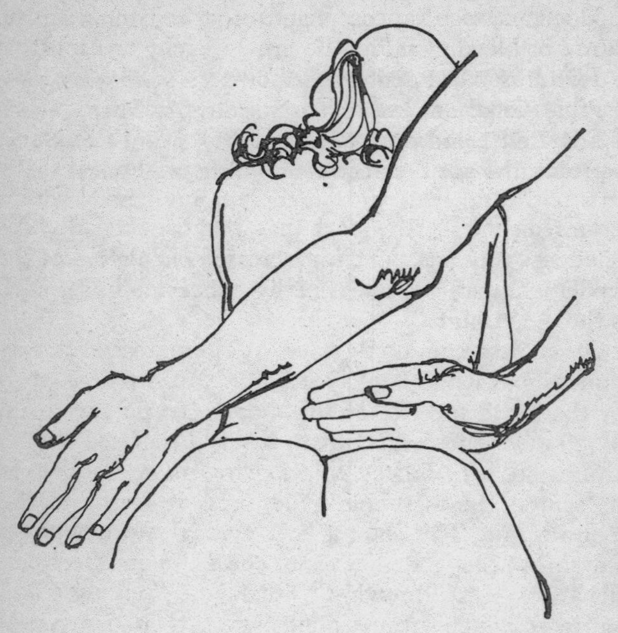

The Chinese and Japanese systems use many additional "thrusting," "pressing," and "tapping" movements, or as Dr. Sidney Zerinsky of the Swedish Institute of Massage in New York calls them, "push-and-pull" movements.

When should a novice not do a general massage?

1. Do not massage a known cardiac patient. (In emergencies cardiac massage may be done by a neophyte for a cardiac arrest.)
2. Don't massage lumps, bumps, or any area suspected of being malignant. Stay away from eruptions, sores, or areas of acute inflammation.

3. If it hurts, *hands off*, unless massage is ordered by a physician or other expert.
4. Don't massage varicose veins, other inflammation of a vein, or blood clots.
5. Don't use deep massage on over-tired muscles; also avoid percussion or kneading on such muscles.
6. Don't do percussion on the spine.
7. Don't massage the abdomen during pregnancy.

4

The Basic "How-To's"

. . . the inability to relax is one of the most widely spread diseases of our civilization, and one of the most infrequently recognized.
*—Flanders Dunbar**

How To Perform a General Massage for Toning, General Improvement of Circulation, and Relaxation

According to the masseur Guy Remsen, President Lyndon Baines Johnson was one of the world's most zealous devotees of body massage as an aid to "unwinding." While still a senator he became addicted to massage following a massive coronary. His doctor told him to "humor his heart" and ordered him to "learn to relax." So he took daily relaxation on the massage table, with an afternoon session in the Senate gym and an evening session at home. When he moved into the White House, he had a nightly massage. A high-ranking American diplomat who traveled with Johnson told how, while in office, Johnson would come home from a day of smiling public appearances, and promptly explode. For two hours he stirred up his

* *The Hygiene of the Quiet Mind*

staff. Then he called in his masseur, and the mood changed almost instantly.

There are similar reports of the use of massage by many presidents and public figures. President Kennedy received massage for his back trouble. Vice President Nelson Rockefeller is said to use massage regularly. *The New York Times* obituary of famed composer Rudolph Friml, who died at the age of ninety-two, mentioned that he was said to have attributed his longevity to sensible diet, rest, sunshine, exercise, and massage. He also used to have his Chinese wife walk barefoot up and down his spinal column—an old Oriental technique.

For a restful, sleep-inducing massage, there are three essentials: regular tempo, light movements, and an unbroken rhythm moving slowly from area to area. Principally, this massage is given by masseurs and masseuses; it is not usually done by physical therapists or those more closely tied to orthodox medicine, where massage is mostly given to treat a specific ailment and the strokes are done in just the area that seem most obviously to be affected.

There are many variations of the general massage; I include some of the more standard strokes. And as I said before, experimentation is very much in order. So let's get started!

General preparation. In describing this massage I will refer to the person being massaged as the "subject," and the person doing the massage as the "masseur," even though the massage can be done by anyone—friend, lover, relative, stranger—not only by a professional masseur or masseuse.

The more relaxed the masseur, the better will be the massage. So it is sometimes helpful first to do relaxation exercises. A good one is the classic yoga relaxation exercise. Lie on the floor on your back in a comfortable position. Turn your thoughts inward, into your body. Part by part, think your body relaxed! Relax your toes, your feet, your soles, your ankles, and so on. It's sometimes good to tense the part you're thinking of first, and then let it relax. After you've done this, lie in place for a few minutes and just think of your breath as it flows in and out, and don't control it. You should be sufficiently relaxed after this to do a good massage.

The atmosphere of the environment in which the massage is done is also very important. The light should be soft. Relaxing music or incense may be used. The room in which the massage is done should be warm, about seventy-five degrees.

Professional masseurs and physical therapists do massage on a regular massage table so they can do the strokes from a standing position, because it is much less strain on them this way. Unless a person is ready to go very deeply into massage, there will probably be no need for such a table. One can improvise. I find it very comfortable to use a thick, warm blanket on the floor. I cover it with fresh, clean, crisp sheets—one under the subject, and one for covering the body areas not being worked. Unfortunately, the massage must then be done in a kneeling or crouching position. To work from a kneeling position takes some adjustment, and it may be a while before it can be done comfortably. If the masseur remembers to work from the entire body and not just the fingers, he will more naturally fall into a comfortable position. Good deep breathing on the part of the masseur will also ultimately lead to a better massage. The energy should flow from the tips of the toes.

On touching. We have inhibitions—all of us—about touching. Unless the massage is being done on someone with whom the masseur is very intimate, the beginning masseur must consciously put aside inhibitions.

The novice might even experience something similar to what Margaret Mead calls "skin-shock." The avoidance, or fear, of touching is quite universal in America. Even barbers these days use electric vibrators to depersonalize the contact of the hand on the scalp. A University of Florida psychologist, Sidney Jourard, who has done some studies on touching, thinks that this confirms psychiatrist R. D. Laing's diagnosis of modern man as "unembodied," and Dr. Jourard sees both encounter groups, in which people are encouraged to touch, and the drug culture as attempts to get back in touch with the body again. I believe the current renewal of interest in massage came about for much the same reason—a reaction to a "skin hunger."

In Western society many of us also confuse the sensual with the sexual, and we suspect that touching must lead naturally to erotic feelings. But this is untrue. All physical contact is not potentially sexual, and one does not have to be sexually involved with everyone he or she touches. It's surprising how many people are unaware of the wide spectrum of feeling available within the realm of what's called "sensual." I even regret the current law pending which will restrict masseurs and masseuses in their practice to only members of the same sex. I realize the intention is probably good, but unfortunately such a restriction could further inhibit and depersonalize us all. I have been massaged myself many times by members of the opposite sex. I am a reasonably normal, reasonably attractive woman, and the men were good-looking and pleasant, but the erotic was not a part of it. And I have seen the same occur in the reverse situation. Granted, an erotic massage between lovers is beautiful, but so too is the lovely sensual joy one feels when being massaged by a member of the opposite sex without sexual involvement.

So I recommend that one relax and abandon himself or herself to the sensual pleasure of touching and being touched.

Anointing with oils. Oil allows the masseurs hands to glide smoothly over the subject's body. It is particularly necessary on the heavy muscles, where there is likely to be resistance, such as on the back and the shoulders, or where there is a lot of hair. On the face and lighter muscles, the body's natural oils are usually sufficient. Still, oil is generally applied once on the entire side being worked, and more is added when required. Vegetable oil, mineral oil, or baby oil may be used. Some masseurs use scents such as lemon oil, clove oil, oil of frangipani, cinnamon oil, or a few drops of perfume. Many of the oils are available at "head shops" or drugstores.

On breathing. "The importance of correct breathing is recognized by all the great teachers," says Gertrude Enelow, and she recalls that the book of Genesis speaks of the mysterious energy, the Spirit (breath) of Life which animates the life process. The Scottish psychoanalyst R. D. Laing claims that if you breathe with the soles of your feet ". . . you may be said to be a man of Tao." He thinks free breathing has helped him to rid himself of sinusitis, rhinitis, and other respiratory difficulties. It is well known by many psychoanalysts that people often hold their breath to suppress anxiety. Ferenczi even had his patients control their breathing as an "activity" during his therapeutic sessions. I mention this here merely to remind anyone about to embark on body work how important breathing is, and I suggest that you think of it from time to time during the massage. If the subject and the masseur breathe freely it will be a better massage. If you have problems, there is one form of yoga called pranayama that concentrates strictly on breathing. I recommend it, or any form of hatha yoga. There are many fine books on the subject, as well as schools throughout the country that teach yoga.

This massage should take about forty-five minutes, and it is an amalgam of many styles, mostly those developed at Esalen. The following directions are to be used only as a guide; all strokes may be used, or only a few, and the order may be varied. Strokes may be done two or three times, or more, depending on the masseur's preference, unless otherwise specified. For greater toning, add deeper strokes and strong kneading; there will still be a sedative effect after the tonic effect wears off.

Now, to begin, shake hands loose to relax them. Rub both hands together to bring up a nice warmth. Start!

There is no set place to begin. For simplicity's sake, you might start at the head. It's also a good starting point inasmuch as the head is too often neglected as a part of the physical body, and it is a common focal point of tension. Massage of the head will produce a new feeling of "lightness," as if weights had been removed.

THE FOREHEAD

1. Kneel at the subject's head. For a few seconds, hold palms lightly against the subject's forehead with fingers at temples. The warmth of the hands is very soothing.

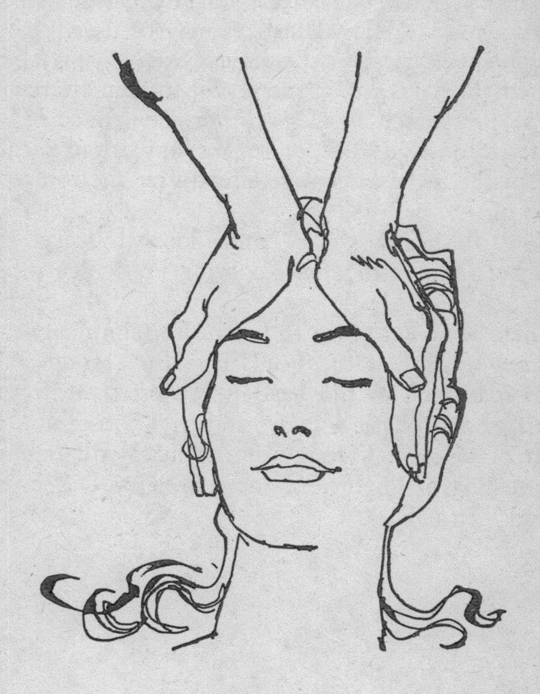

Instead of using the palms, the masseur might hold the thumbs at the center of the forehead with fingertips out toward the temples.

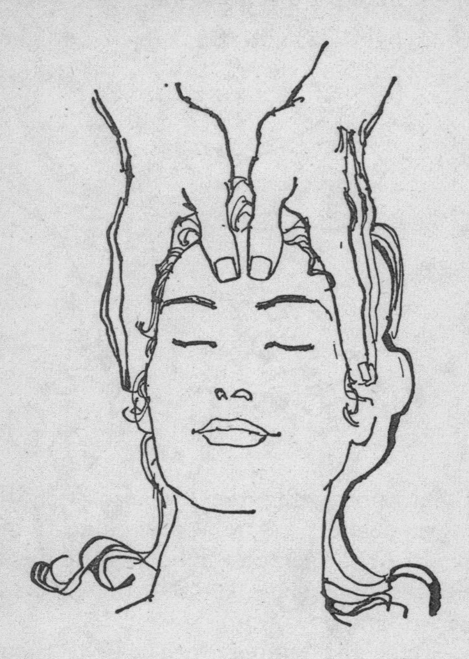

2. In addition to 1, or instead of it, simply press with both hands, one on top of each other, with moderate pressure for a few seconds.

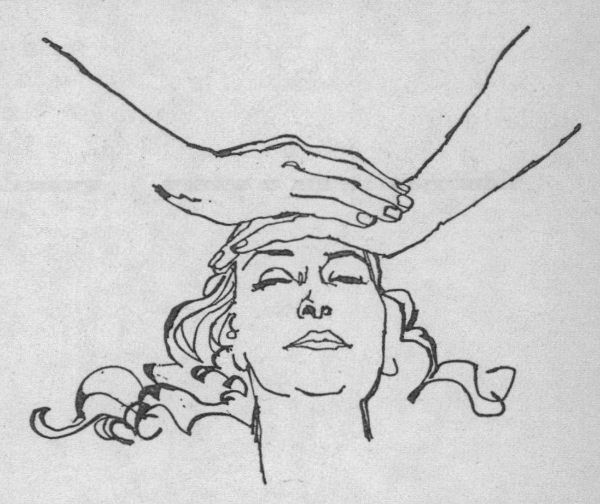

3. Start massaging the forehead with the thumbs, using moderate pressure and working from the center outward. At the temples, move a little downward, and, barely touching, slide hands to the center again. Continue working downward.

4. Stroke the temples with a light circular motion. This may be done with thumbs held at the center of the forehead.

THE EYES

5. With all fingertips, forefinger, or thumb, stroke the upper lid, moving outward toward the temple. Use enough pressure so that the eyeballs are palpable under the fingertips. Repeat for the lower lid.

6. With both forefingers, find the bony rim of the eye sockets where they connect with the nose. Exert pressure there for a few seconds. Then slowly press all along the upper and lower rims. This is a variation of

the Oriental pressure massage, and it is supposedly good for the sinuses.

CHEEKS AND NOSE

7. This is optional, but it is very good for stimulating and loosening the face muscles. Flattened hands are applied to the cheeks, fingers pointing to the chin. The flesh of the cheeks is slowly rotated so the subject's lips move up and down.

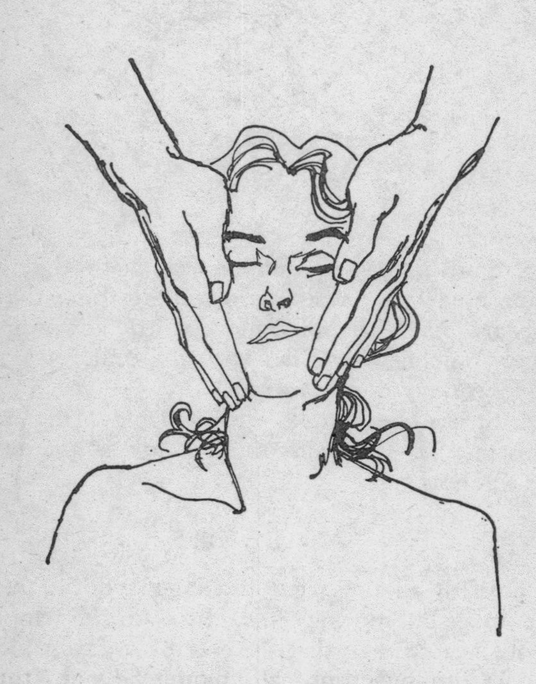

8. Stroke outward with the fingertips, following the cheekbones to the temples.

9. When at the lower edge of the cheekbones, rest awhile, pressing hard along the lower edges in a circular motion. This helps to relieve tension of the face.

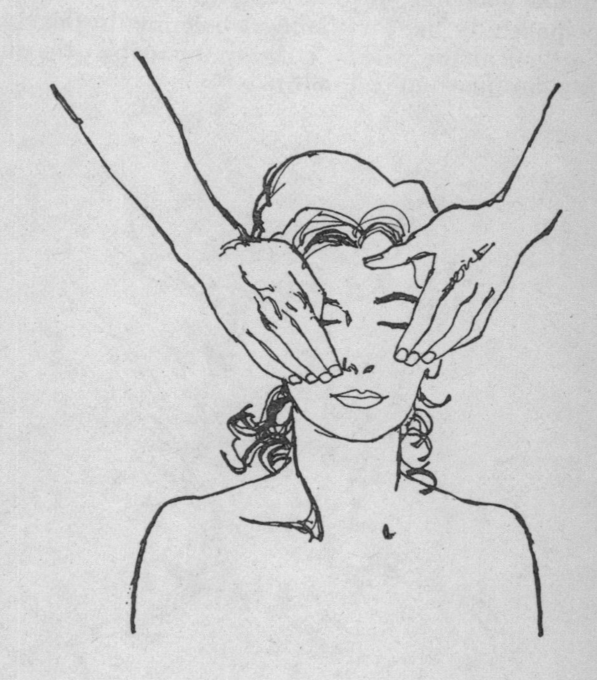

10. With fingertips at temples, and thumbs touching the tip of the nose, move upward with the thumbs on the nose, using a firm kneading movement. At the bridge of the nose, pause, and apply pressure in the hollows where the nose meets the eye socket.

BOTTOM HALF OF FACE

11. Use a series of horizontal strokes on the bottom of the face, as was done on the forehead.

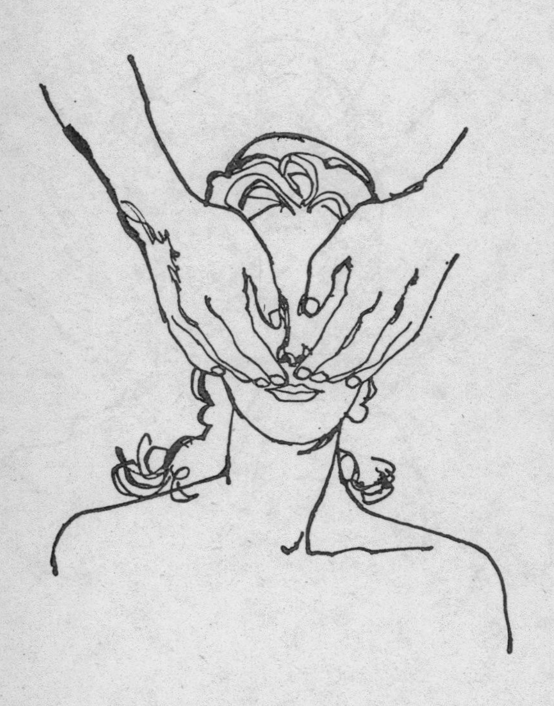

12. Grasp the edge of the chin with both hands, holding it between the fingers and thumb. Slowly follow the edges of the jaw to the ears. On return strokes, use a light gliding movement.

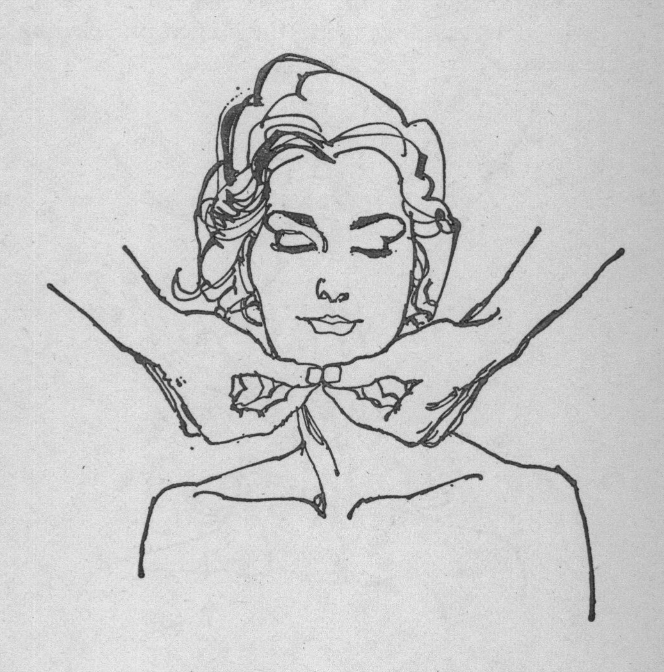

THE EARS

13. There are many ways to massage the ears. They may be done one at a time or together. The ears are usually ignored by physical therapists or professional masseurs, but they are done in the Esalen-style massage. And why not? Are they not parts of the body too? A new life and vitality may be felt when they are pressed, so try stroking with the fingertips, exerting some pressure.

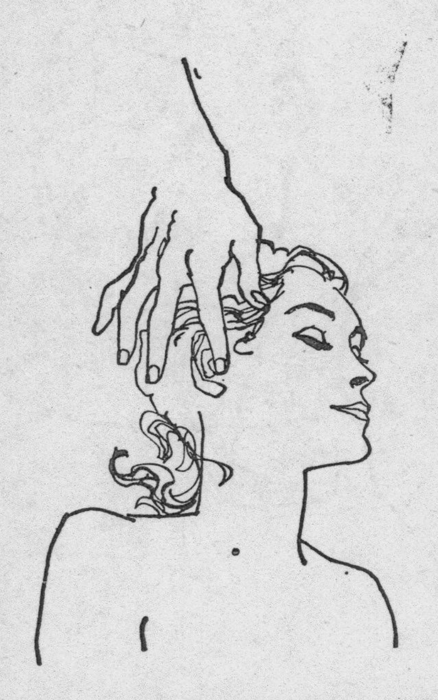

14. Try pinching the outer rim of the ear and earlobe, then letting the fingers glide around the edges.

15. Do some strokes just below the ears where the skull meets the jaw.

THE NECK

We all experience a great deal of tension in this area, and the region of the shoulders and upper back. The relief felt when this area is massaged is magnificent.

16. Slide both hands, with palms up, under the subject's neck, keeping the backs of the hands on the table. The area is worked as far down as the hands can reach, and up to the bottom of the skull. Tapping or vibrating movements are used. Pressure should be exerted.

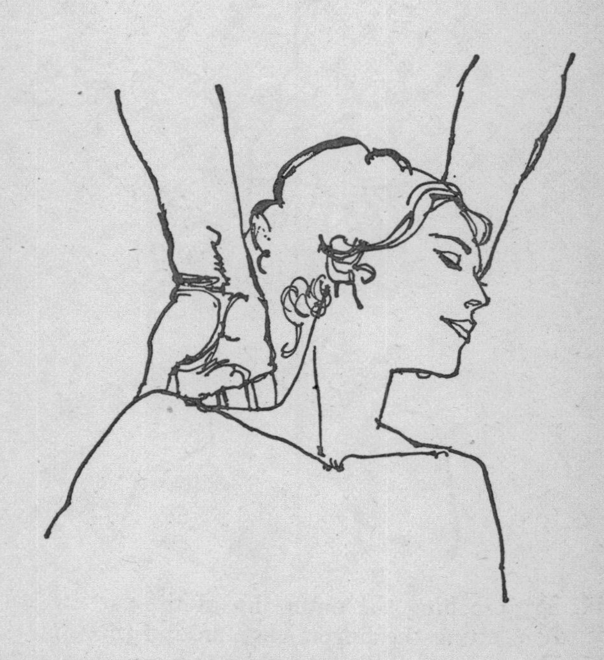

17. With hands under the subject's head, the masseur lifts the head gently and turns it to one side, allowing it to rest in one hand. If the subject tries to "help," remind him to let go of his tension. The masseur, must do the lifting. Now stroke the shoulder, neck, and back with the entire hand, cupped, using fingertips in areas where the whole hand cannot reach. Pressure may be applied in the neck and back area. Circular movements are also good in this region. Repeat on the other side.

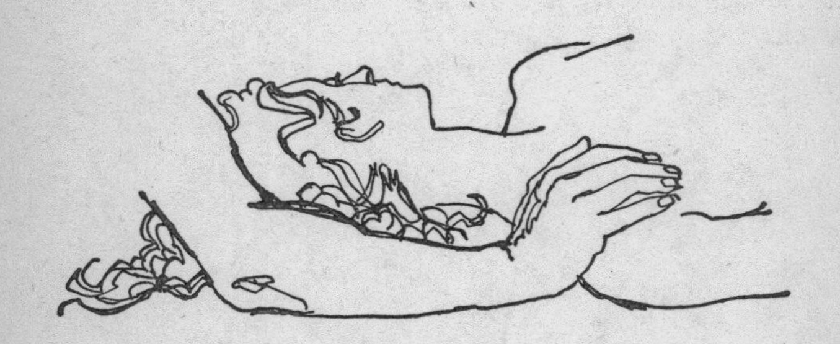

THE SCALP

18. With the head still turned, use cupped fingers stretched out like claws to massage the scalp. Use enough pressure so that the bones can be felt beneath the scalp. Work the entire area. Repeat on the other side.

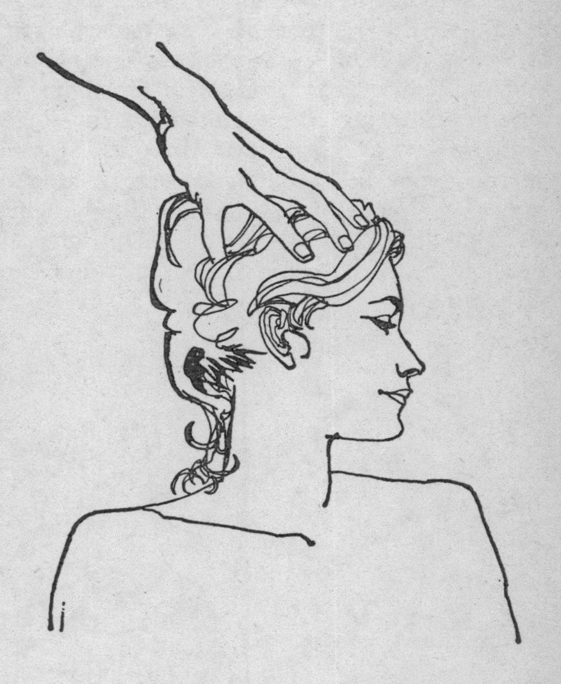

THE TORSO (FRONT)

19. Move the subject's head back in place. This is called the "main stroke." To start, hold hands together in the middle of the chest, palms down and cupped to fit the contours of the body. The fingers are pointing toward the subject's feet. Glide both hands forward, using pressure on the chest and a lighter touch on the stomach. At the bottom of the stomach, separate hands and move them to the subject's sides. Grasp the side of the subject's body and pull firmly up to the armpits. Then swing hands around so the fingertips point to the center. This is repeated about six times, and the masseur may keep coming back to it after other strokes are completed. It can be varied by bringing the hands around the shoulders or the back of the head and neck when the hands reach the armpits and another stroke is about to be started.

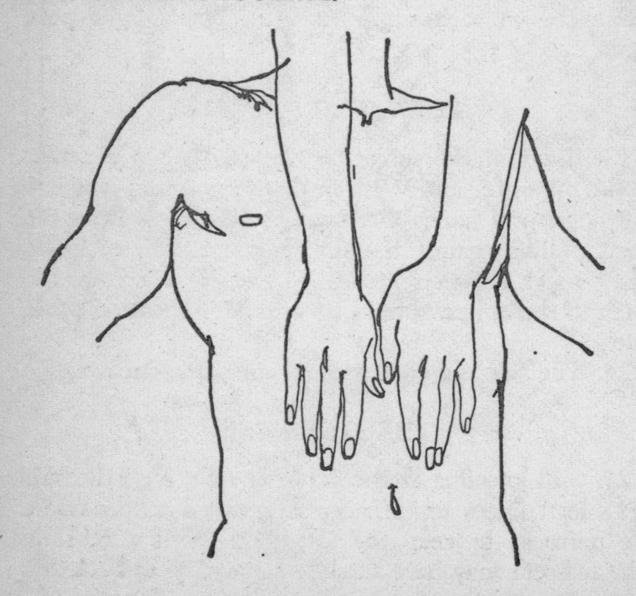

20. This is a variation of the main stroke, and it also helps restore circulation in the chest area. The masseur moves to the subject's waist, facing the head, and places both hands flat on the body, fingers pointing inward. Pressure is then applied and hands move upwards, across the abdomen and chest. At the neck, the hands slide lightly down along the subject's side to the starting point.

21. Masseurs do not usually massage a woman's breasts, mostly out of prudishness. The Esalen-type massage includes it. Use a gentle stroking motion with cupped hands. Whether to do it or not should depend largely on the subject. If the subject is "uptight," don't.

22. Kneeling at the subject's head, make hands into fists. Place both fists at the middle of the chest just below the collarbone and then slide them out across the chest to the sides, following the ribs. Go into the hollows between each rib individually, using light pressure.

THE TORSO (SIDES)

23. Kneel at the subject's waist and reach across it to the opposite side. With fingertips pointing down to the floor, pull hands alternately straight up from the floor, pulling against the subject's side. There should be no break between strokes. The entire side from the thigh to the armpit should be worked. Repeat on other side.

24. The side is a good area for kneading strokes.

THE STOMACH

25. Still kneeling at the subject's side, raise the subject's legs, knees up. If necessary, put a pillow under the buttocks to keep the knees up without tension. The masseur may have to slide subject's feet back and

forth until a comfortable position is found. With the palm of one hand, little circles are made, moving clockwise from the waist around to the pelvic bone, and back. The masseur could also add the other hand and have it follow the first one. Put the subject's knees back in place.

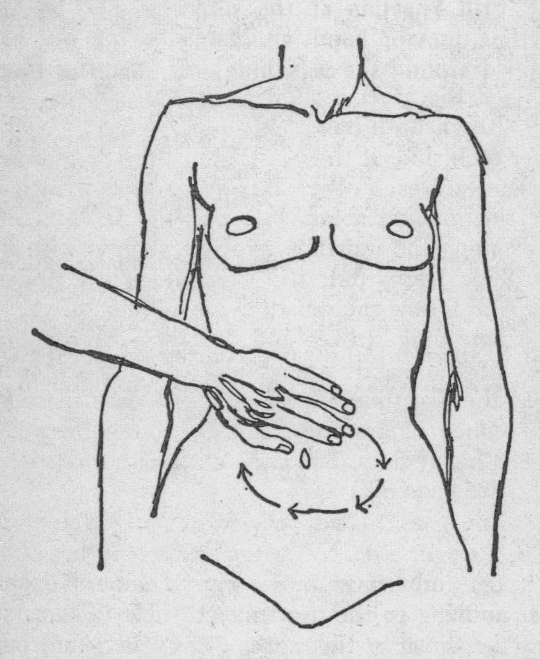

26. This stroke is particularly good if the subject is constipated, as it drains the colon to relieve the body of waste matter. Hold fingers closely together and move over the lower abdomen, following the imagined coils of the intestine. The palm of the other hand follows the first hand.

Physical therapists work the colon somewhat differently, using a kneading stroke with the fingertips of one hand, reinforced by the other one on top of it.

27. The masseur may also do deep-stroking over the abdominal region, using one hand on top of the other, working over the ribs and then down to the abdomen. Kneading may also be done in this region.

THE WAIST

28. Still kneeling at the subject's side, stroke the waistline, moving hands alternately. While one hand is wrapped around the waistline with fingertips touching the floor, the other is sliding across the waist.

29. Reach both hands under the subject's back, one under each side, at the waist. Palms are up, and fingers point toward each other. Fingertips should reach to either side of the spine, but not *on* the spine. Slide hands along the waistline, pressing slightly with fingertips. Slide hands out, still pressing lightly under the back, and follow the waistline onto the stomach.

30. Kneading strokes and "sawing"—or moving the edges of the hands alternately, as if sawing wood—across the waistline are thought by some masseurs to help reduce inches from the waistline. I'm not convinced that it does, but it does at least tone the muscles. (See page 32.)

THE FOREARMS

31. One arm must be done at a time. To get the blood moving to the heart, use a basic massage stroke from the wrist to the upper arm. Hands are cupped over the subject's arm, side by side, thumbs touching. Firm pressure is applied as the hands glide up the arm. At the top, one hand moves over the top of the shoulder, and the other hand moves down inside the arm. Then both hands pull lightly down the arm, one on the outside, the other on the inside. At the end, before another stroke is begun masseur may continue the stroke down to the subject's hand and lightly press it between his own hands. (See following page.)

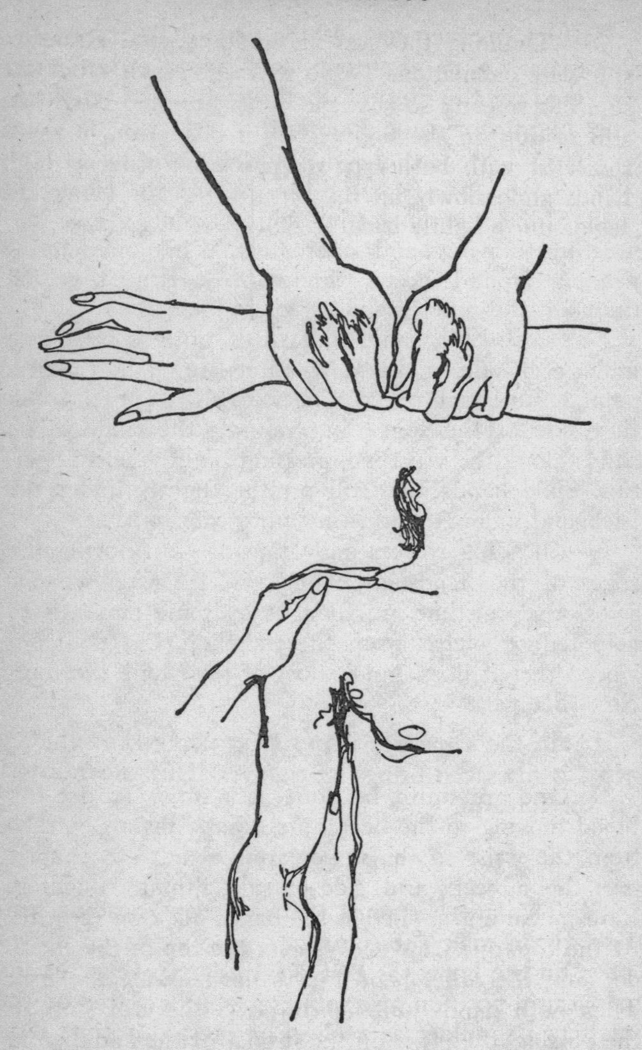

32. "Draining the arm" is another good stroke to stimulate circulation. To do it, the masseur raises the subject's forearm so that the upper arm and elbow are still resting on the floor. Then a ring is made about the wrist with both hands, lightly squeezing as both hands glide slowly up the forearm. At the elbow the hands move lightly back.

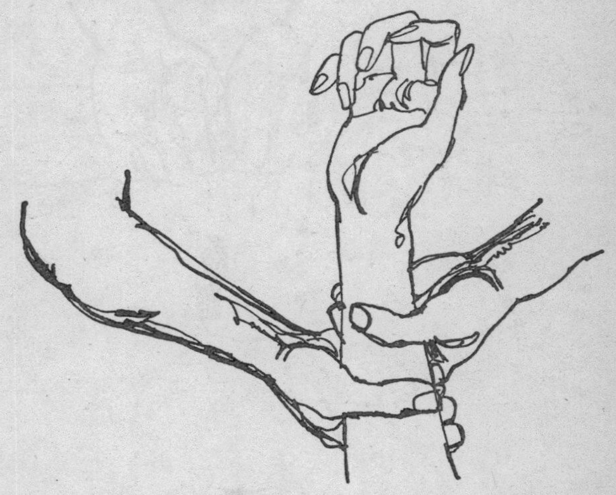

33. In the same position, the inside of the subject's wrist is massaged using the thumbs. This is continued up the forearm.

THE UPPER ARM

34. This area responds well to heavy kneading, particularly in male subjects. Care must be taken not to press on the bones, as that may hurt. To keep the upper arm in position, the subject's hand is placed on the masseur's shoulder as a cheek is pressed against it to hold it in place.

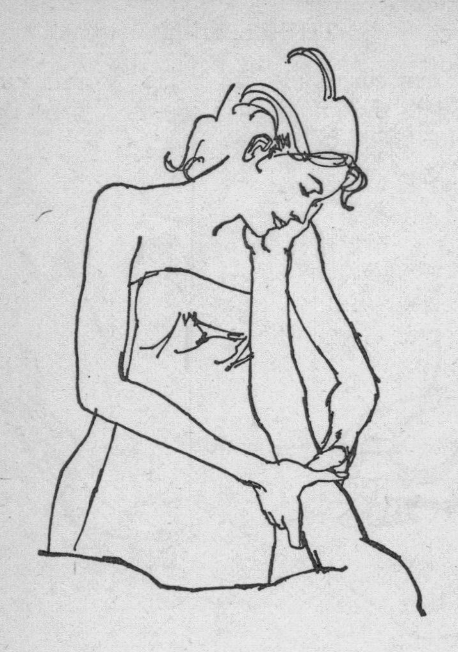

35. and 36. The same basic stroke and "draining" stroke are done here as on the forearm.

37. Tossing the subject's arm back and forth a few times between the masseur's hands is experienced as quite invigorating, but the masseur must take care not to break the relaxed mood with this movement.

38. It is a lovely flourish to brush up and down the subject's arm very lightly, like a caress, with the fingertips.

THE ELBOW

39. The masseur holds the subject's arm upright again, and with the knuckles of the other hand lightly massages the inside of the elbow joint.

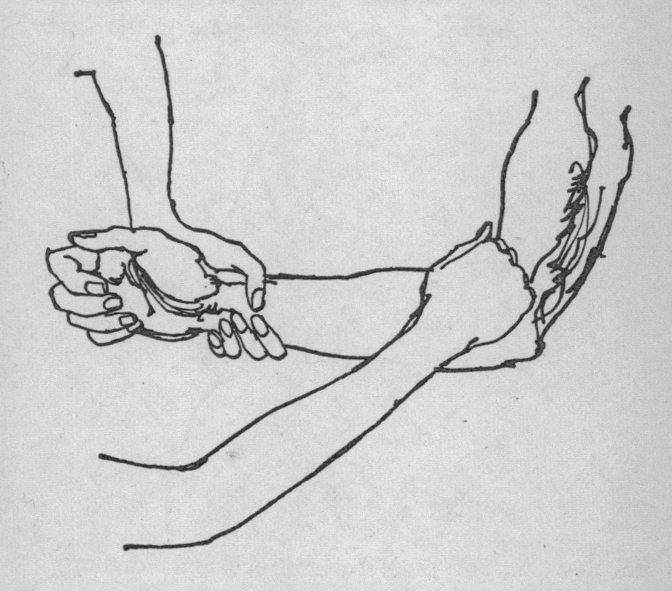

40. Then, holding the forearm with one hand, the masseur works the elbow with the tips of the fingers, making tiny circles.

THE HANDS

41. Holding the subject's hand, palm up, in one hand, the masseur uses the other hand to massage the palm with knuckles, moving in small circles. The same thing is also done with the thumbs. Moderate pressure may be used here. This also may be done on the inside of the wrist with less pressure.

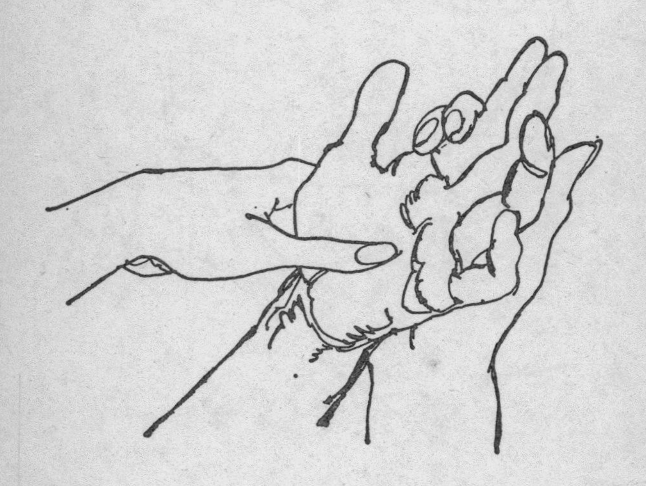

42. Use the same circular massage for the back of the hand, moving up onto the wrist. Try to feel all the little bones on the subject's hand. The masseur may also try kneading here, moving in little circles with the thumbs.

43. Masseur slowly runs fingers (or thumb) down subject's hand along the ridges between the tendons. These are the cords on the back of the hand that run from the wrist to the knuckles.

THE FINGERS

44. Grasp subject's fingers one by one, exerting a slight pulling movement, turning as one would a cork-screw. (drawing #27)

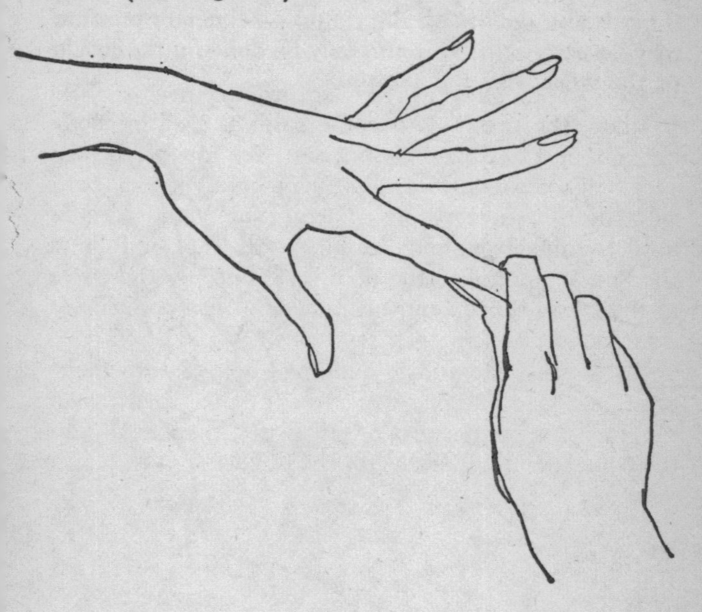

45. A beautiful finale: masseur holds subject's hand sandwiched between his own, pausing and concentrating only on the breath as it moves in and out.

THE LEGS (CALVES)

46. Masseur kneels at subject's feet, to the side of the leg being worked. The main stroke, which stimulates circulation, is the same as the one done for the fore arms. (See page 57.) Legs are done one at a time. Both hands are cupped, fingers together. Masseur then

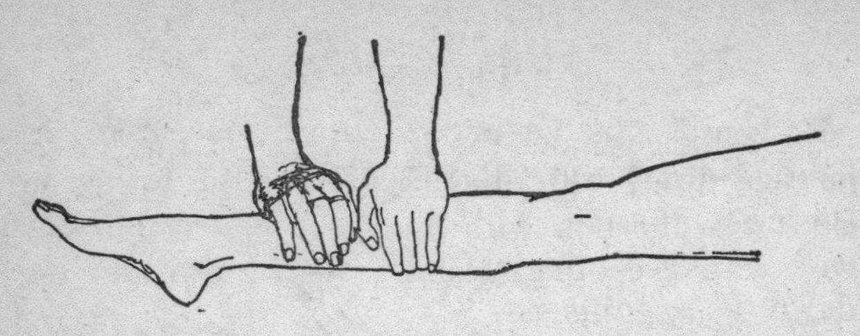

lets his hands glide up the leg, leaning over slightly to allow the pressure to come from the entire body and not just the hands alone. At the top of the leg the hands separate and glide very lightly down both sides of the subject's leg. The outside hand reaches until the fingertips find the hip bone. Here it follows the line of the hip to the floor, as it outlines the curve of the bone. Movements are timed so that both hands move down the leg together.

47. As with the arms, "draining" helps improve circulation. To do it, first work to the knee, then stroke the knee (as in the next few strokes), then finally do the same "draining" stroke for the thighs.

THE KNEES

48. Massage under the lower edge of the kneecap, pressing firmly with thumbs. Follow the furrow in a clockwise direction with one hand and counterclockwise with the other. Hands cross at top and move down the opposite side.

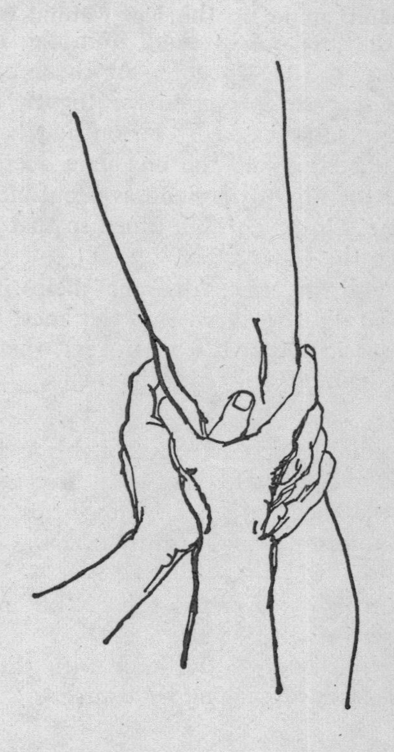

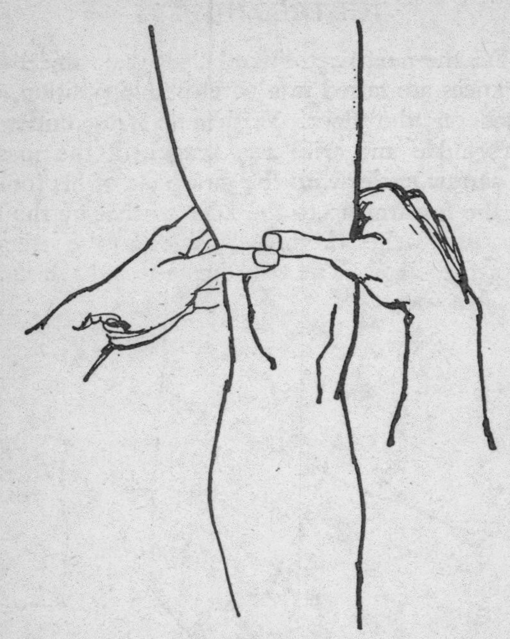

49. Kneading is very effective in this area. One way to knead is to rest the heels of both hands at the lower border of the knee and with the fingertips at the upper border. Thumbs may glide lightly over the entire kneecap.

50. Drum lightly over the top of the kneecap with tips of fingers of both hands.

51. Rub the sides of the knee with the fingers of both hands at once, making wide circles.

THE LEGS (UPPER)

52. For the next two strokes, place the subject's legs so the knees are raised in a comfortable position, with the feet on the floor. With one arm under the subject's ankle and with fists clenched, the masseur makes narrow circles with the underside of his forearm, sliding the forearm up to the knee so that by the time the masseur reaches the top of the calf he is using the crook of the elbow. The masseur moves down the leg in the same way.

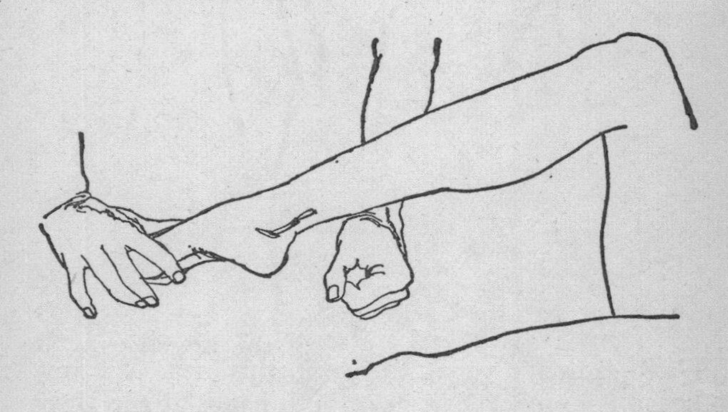

53. The following is called "rolling," and it may also be done for the arm. To do it, palms are placed on either side of the thigh where it meets the knee. Fingers point to the subject's head. Hands are moved back and forth up the thigh and down again in a rolling motion, as if rolling a cigarette. Put subject's legs back in position again.

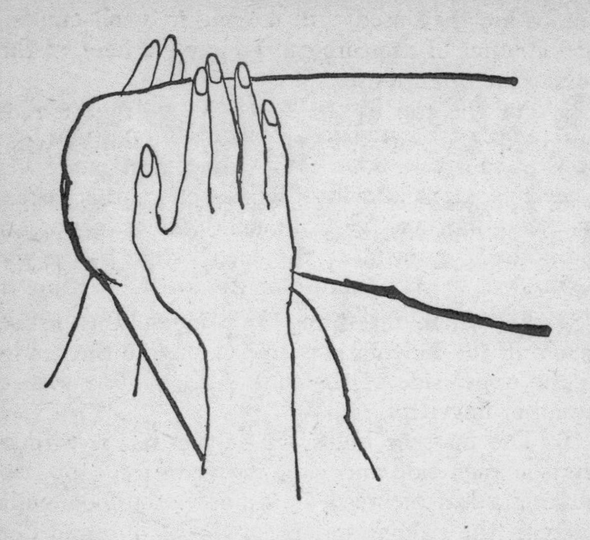

THE THIGH

54. A fine area for kneading strokes.

55. To end, brush the leg with the fingertips from toes to hip with long rhythmic strokes.

THE FEET

Most people neglect their feet; they wear bad shoes, and they stand improperly tipped over onto the balls of their feet. Yet there is an entire system of massage, called zone therapy, or reflexology, based solely on massage of the feet. Zone therapists think that the foot is a "map" of the entire body and there is a reflex area there relative to every part or organ.

56. The masseur may need to prop the subject's foot up on a pillow or place it in his lap. A fist is made with one hand, and small circles are etched over the entire bottom of the foot with the knuckles. The

thumbs are then used, still moving in small circles. A good amount of pressure can be applied here, as these muscles are often tense.

57. For the top of the foot, the masseur uses the thumbs in the same way as he did on the bottom of the foot.

58. The ankle is worked with the thumbs or fingertips of both hands. Spend some time massaging with fingertips around the ankle bone, working into the crevices.

59. As when massaging the hand, the masseur presses in the indentations that lie beside the tendons on the upper side of the foot. This is done with the thumb or fingertips.

60. The masseur holds the subject's foot with one hand on each side and with the thumb on top. As if breaking a loaf of bread, he squeezes the foot, pulling out with the palmar surface of the thumb and down over the rest of the fingers. Very slowly, the top of the masseur's hand moves from the middle of the foot out to either edge.

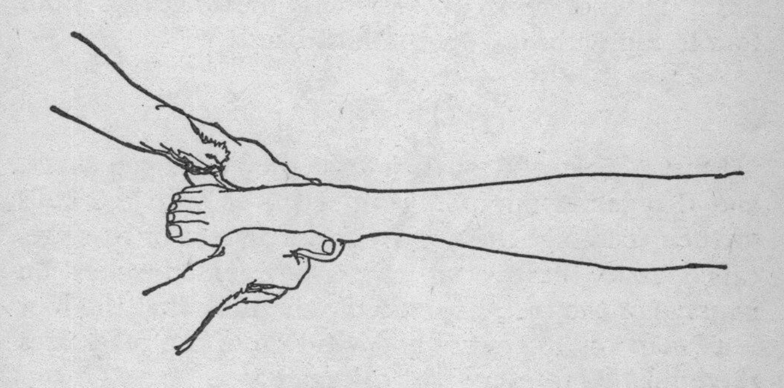

61. The foot is particularly amenable to kneading. The heel of the hand is used, and pressure is applied under the arch. (See following page.)

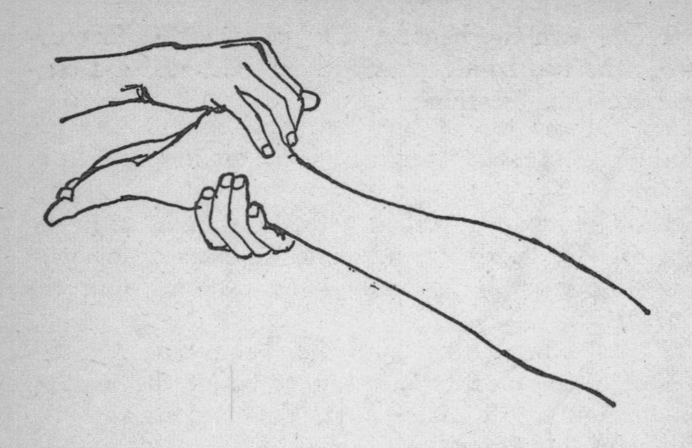

THE TOES

62. Work the toes, one by one, pulling in a cork-screw motion. Flex them, stroke them, rotate them—anything to bring life and vitality to this neglected area.

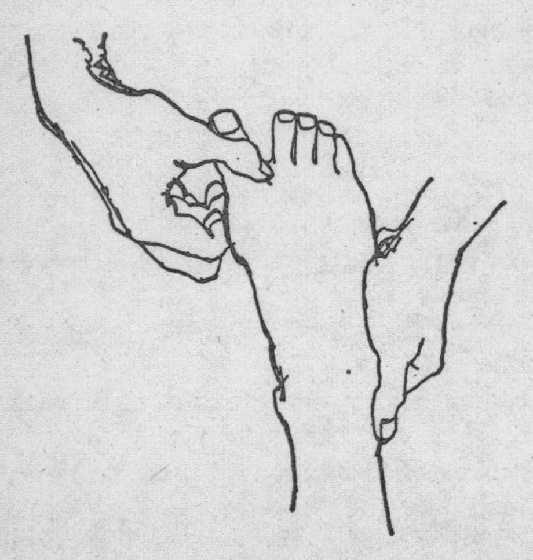

63. As with the hand, end by pressing the foot between the two hands, pausing a few seconds, and concentrating on breathing.

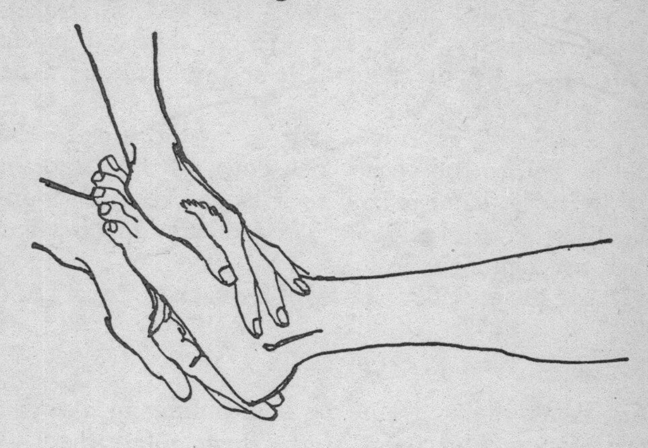

THE BACK

The masseur asks the subject to turn over, and one hand is kept in contact with the subject's body as he moves. Spread some oil over the back.

THE LEGS (BACK)

64. The same main stroke is done here as on the front of the legs. More pressure may be used on the back of the legs.

65. As on the front of the leg, the "draining" stroke may be done.

66. Kneading is also appropriate for the back of the legs.

67. A stroke called "wringing" may be done, which is very much like the "Indian burn" you may have done as a child. To do it, the masseur cups both hands around the leg at the ankle and moves up the leg as if wringing clothes.

68. Use balls of the thumbs to massage the thick muscles of the calf.

69. Beginning at the inside of the thigh just past the knees, "pull" up the leg in slow vertical strokes, keeping the palms in contact with the skin and fingers pointing toward the floor. The return stroke is done very lightly.

70. "Raking" is a superb stroke for the back of the legs, as well as the entire back down to the buttocks. To do it, the hand is held so it looks like a rake. Unlike all other strokes, "rake" in a downward direction when massaging the leg.

71. At the end, flex the leg as far back as it will go.

THE BUTTOCKS

72. The muscles here respond to strong kneading. Do regular stroking with the fingertips. Do this systematically.

73. Make small circles with the fingertips across and down the side of the buttocks.

74. Try to find the hollows between the two large muscles—the gluteus medius and the gluteus maximus—which is about an inch to the side of the center of the buttocks. If the exact spot can't be found, any spot in the general area is good enough. Exert firm pressure with knuckles.

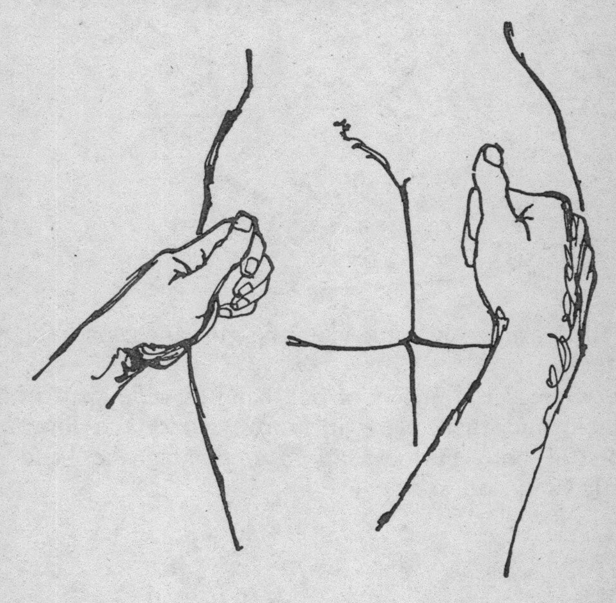

Then use the heel of the hand in the same area. Make a vibrating motion by shaking the entire arm as fast as possible.

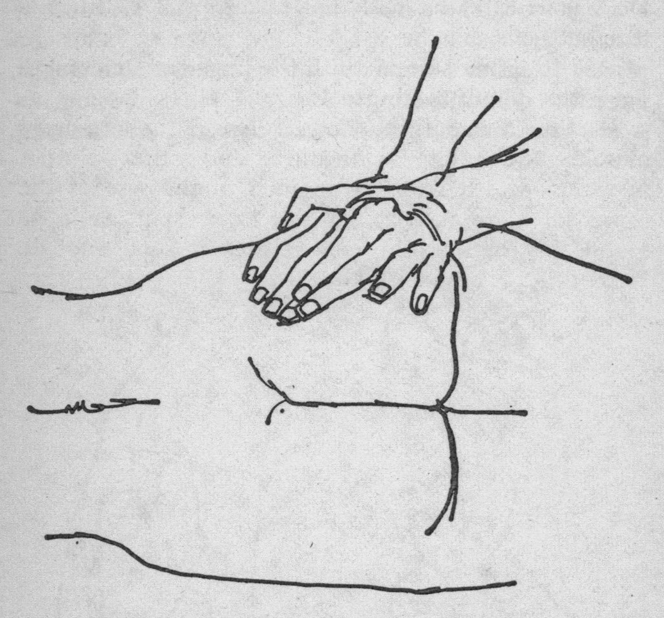

75. Continue the same vibrating movement over the buttocks.

76. Spread the fingers of one hand as wide apart as possible and then place it firmly against the lower slopes of both buttocks at once, shaking the hand lightly from side to side.

THE BACK

77. The masseur can work from either the subject's head or foot. These directions require that he kneel at the subject's side or straddle the subject. Palms are placed to either side of the spine, but not touching it, fingertips pointing inward to spine. Press, moving upward from the waist to the shoulders. At the armpits,

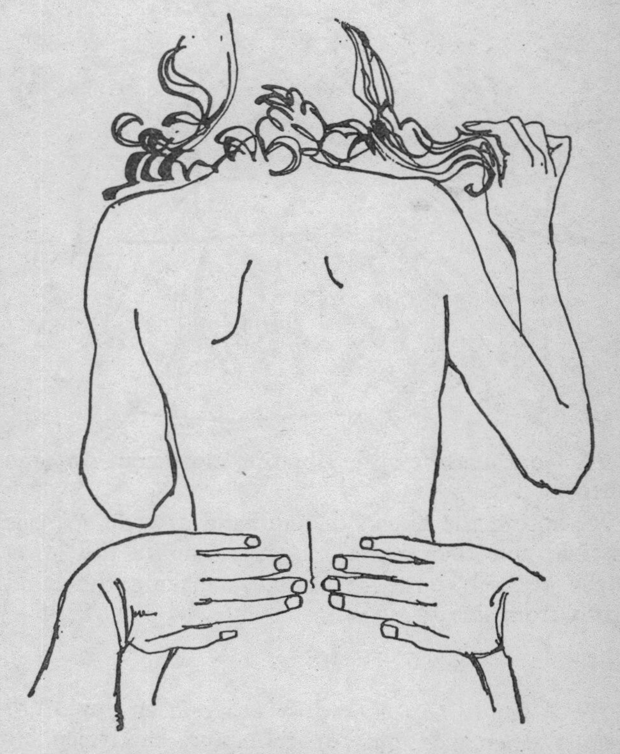

gently separate hands till they touch the floor, then back, lightly touching the subject's torso, to the waist. Then move down along the side of the hips and return, using less pressure. This stroke can be repeated at intervals after others are done.

78. This stroke is similar to the previous one. The masseur starts at the lower back (sacrum), fingers pointing to the head, thumbs crossed to give added strength. The hands move up on each side of the spine with firm pressure. At the neck, the hands separate and stroke over the top of the shoulder and down the sides of the back to the waist.

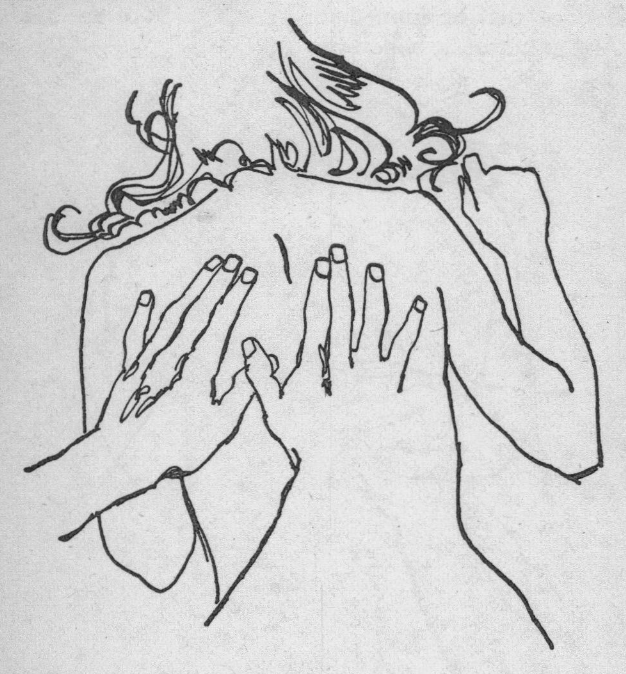

79. *A law to be followed*: Massage in an upward direction when massaging *on* the spine, and when out about an inch, stroke *down* the spine. Given that this rule is followed, there's room for improvisation when massaging the back.

80. Here's a stroke that takes that law nicely into account. It's called the "rocking horse." To do it, masseur places one hand on the spine, palm down, fingers pointing to the subject's head. The other hand is placed horizontally on top of it. Hands move up the spine, pressure exerted by the heel of the hand. On the return stroke, the bottom hand is lifted slightly so it no longer touches the spine, and the tops of the second and third fingers are pressed deep into the two hollows that lie immediately to the side of the spine. At the buttocks, widen the fingers.

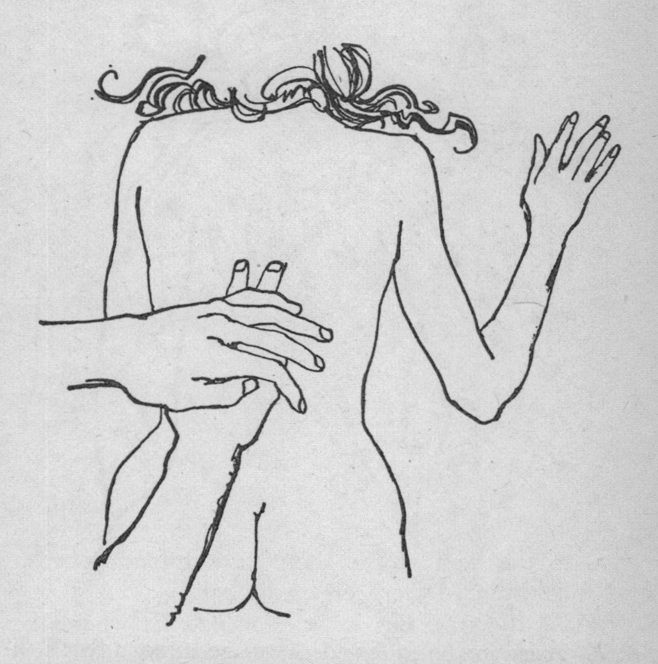

81. Do "pulling" along the sides of the torso, as when working the front of the torso.

82. Kneading is very good for the upper back, a high-tension area.

83. For the shoulders, press up from just beneath the shoulderblades with flattened hands, fingers pointing to subject's head. Slide lightly over the shoulder blades and curl fingers over the ridge of the shoulders. As this is done, the heels of the hands are pressed up-

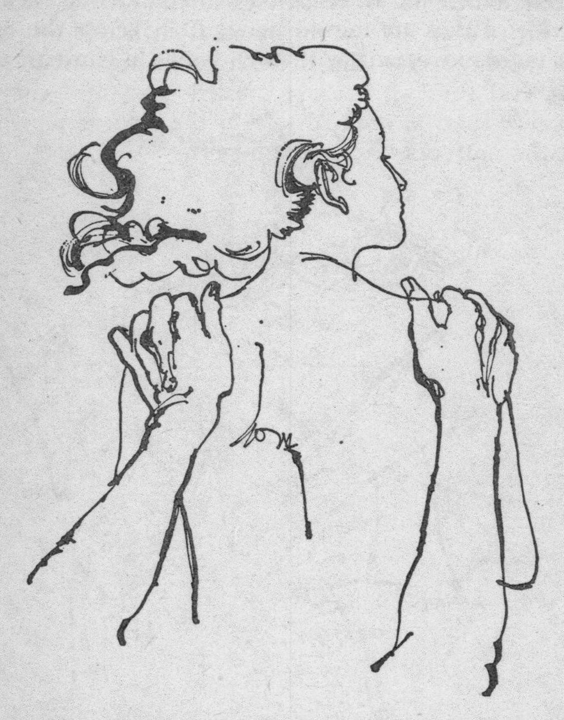

ward so the flesh of the shoulder is folded between the fingertips and the heels of the hands.

84. At the trapezius muscles, which lie where the neck meets the shoulders, kneading is done with two hands. One hand is placed flat over the area. The other hand is placed over the first. Small circular movements are done systematically over the entire region of the neck and shoulders.

85. Palms are placed over the tops of the shoulders, with thumbs spread. Muscles are picked up as the hands move inward toward the neck and cervical region.

86. The "wringing" stroke is applicable here, and it is done much the same as it was done for the back of the legs. Palms are moved horizontally across the back in a rapid movement, with both hands in constant motion.

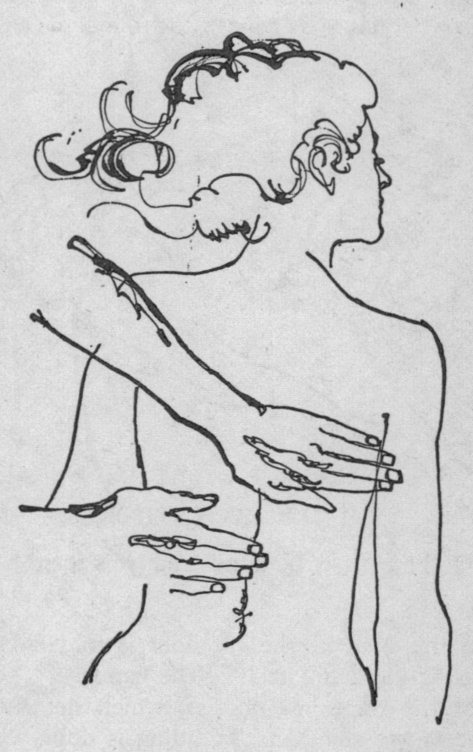

87. The undersides of both forearms are placed straight across the back near the waist. Forearms start out close together, and hands are raised. Slowly forearms are spread apart, with hard pressure, until one arm is at the top of the back and the other is at the thighs. Arms are lifted, lightly touching and returned to the starting position, and the stroke is repeated. To repeat this for the subject's far side, the masseur shifts his weight while remaining in the same position. It may also be done diagonally, working at an angle.

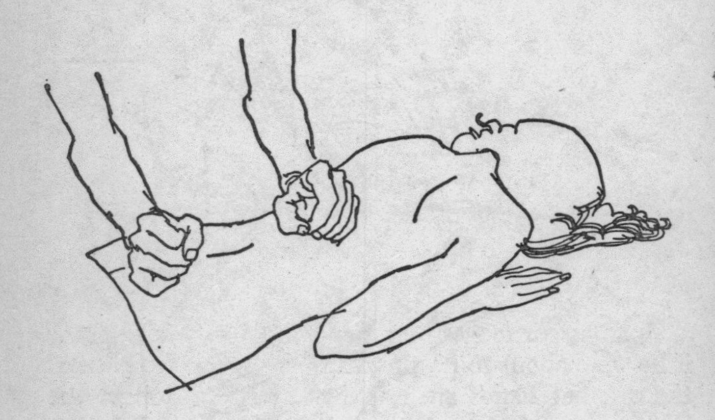

FULL-LENGTH STROKES

88. "Raking" may be done exactly as for the back of the leg.

89. "Hacking" is very invigorating. To do it, drum the outer edges of the hands lightly but rapidly around the spine, starting at the top and working downward. Continue moving down one leg and then up and down the other.

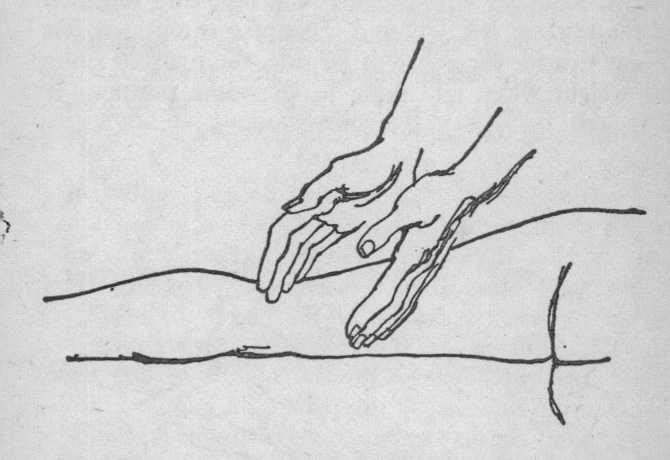

90. Masseur moves both hands up on the leg, just as if he were about to do the main stroke for the back of the leg, but hands are not divided at the top of the leg. Instead, hands continue without a break right over the buttocks and up one side of the back. Hands are separated at the shoulderblades and finally brought, heels first, back down the sides of the legs to the ankle, lightly touching. Don't move on the spine.

TO END

91. Using both hands at once, do a series of feather-light strokes, brushing up and down subject's body from the neck to the feet, using only the fingertips. If the skin is still oily, apply alcohol or witch hazel.

Subject should remain in position, not moving, relaxing.

On Erotic Massage. The mind is the first and foremost erogenous zone, so any massage can be an erotic massage if both partners wish it.

General massage is a good prelude to eroticism; it also has the advantage that it relaxes a person. Contrary to what one may think, the secret of an erotic massage is not necessarily a massage of the genitals, for there are many other erogenous areas throughout the body. These vary to some extent from person to person, as lovers soon discover if their spirits are open and loving.

To arouse sexuality, take turns doing a general massage—which, by the way, should include more featherlight strokes than usual. Then, together, stroke erogenous areas other than the genitals. Generally, these are located on the *insides* of the body: the insides of the thighs, insides of the arms, the armpits, inside of the buttocks, the navel, in the middle of the lower back, inside the ears, in the palms, the nipples, the inner sections of the toes, the nape of the neck, the back of the legs. You may substitute the breath for the hands. Finally, massage the genitals with light pressure with the fingertips, moving in a circular pattern. One needn't try to arouse a lover; it will happen.

More on Swedish Massage. Swedish massage includes most of the general massage strokes given in this book, only in Sweden the massage is often done in a sauna bath or a steam room. The treatment sometimes is enhanced by stroking the back with willow branches or palm leaves. For a makeshift steam room, turn on the hot water in the shower and let the tub fill. Keep the door closed. For facial massage, use hot towels followed by cold towels. Finish up the treatment with an alcohol rub.

5

Your Body Loves You

Talk about a man's individuality and character:
it's the way he uses himself.
*—F. Matthias Alexander**

Many of the strokes mentioned in the last two chapters can be modified for self-massage. The facial strokes, the shoulder strokes, the strokes of the calves and the feet, and those of the arms and hands are particularly easy to adapt. But there are also some other strokes that are uniquely suited for a person to do on himself or herself, because they can be done with a minimum of tension of the arms—one of the major stumbling blocks to a good, relaxing self-massage.

There are also small special advantages to self-massage. It can be done repeatedly whenever needed; it's almost like having your own masseur "on call." These strokes are ideal for toning and awakening a person from a dull feeling, or feelings of lethargy or tension. Many of them we do automatically. I find that when I'm tired from hunching over my typewriter, I do a few choice strokes. My tired eyes also respond to some yoga techniques I've learned. It is advisable for anyone doing self-massage to study yoga; it can have excellent benefits.

The following is a ten-minute massage incorporating

* from *The Resurrection of the Body*, New York, Delta, 1969

yoga, variations of the Esalen-type massage, and other standard methods. It is done lying or sitting on a bed. I also include a tub-bath self-massage; this provides the best possible relaxation, and if done in a warm, soapy bath, the suds may be used as a lubricant.

A Self-Massage

THE FACE

1. You may do the facial strokes described in the last chapter that you can modify for self massage. For forehead strokes, use the fingertips instead of the thumbs.

2. Rest the palms of both hands under your cheekbones, fingertips pointing upward toward the scalp. Move palms up so you can feel your cheekbones

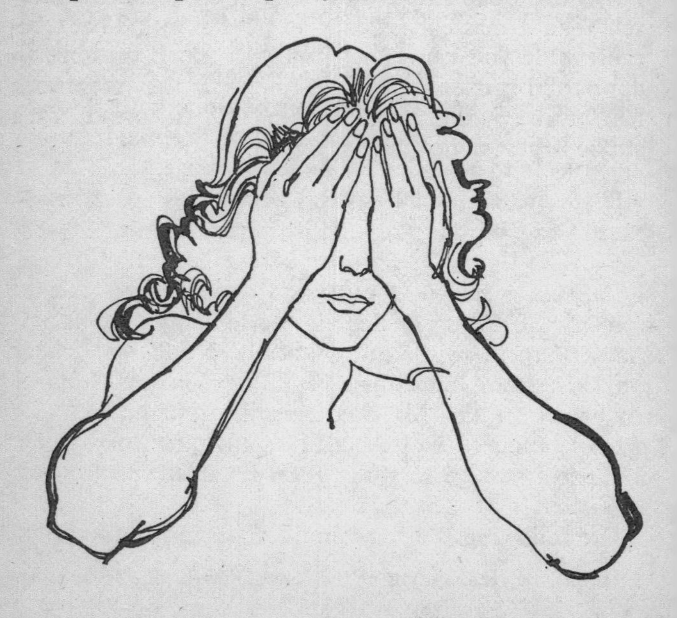

underneath your hands. Work around the entire bone to the temples in this way. Then, with fingertips closed, stroke cheeks and forehead from the center out to the temples.

THE EYES

3. This is a yoga exercise that I find helps when my eyes are tired or strained. I do it many times a day. First, rub hands together to raise a nice warmth. Then place palms over the closed eyes with fingertips touching the hairline. Rest hands there. Then move hands down so the fingertips touch the eyelids. Stroke eyelids outward toward the temples, using the closed fingertips or just one finger.

THE SCALP

4. Here's one stroke that you can do better on yourself than a masseur is likely to do for you. That's because only you can know just how much pressure to apply, and masseurs are often timid lest they mess your hair. Rub vigorously with your fingers spread. This stroke is best done while sitting.

THE NECK

5. Remain seated. Press as hard as you can at either side of the spine. Move in a circular, vibrating motion as far down as you can reach on the back. Do the same for the shoulders. You may also do kneading with the

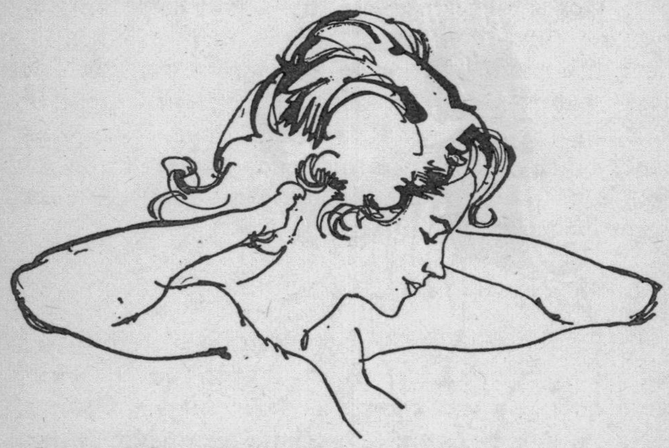

palms and fingertips in the same region.

6. Upward strokes on the front of the neck are thought to erase potential lines and sagging.

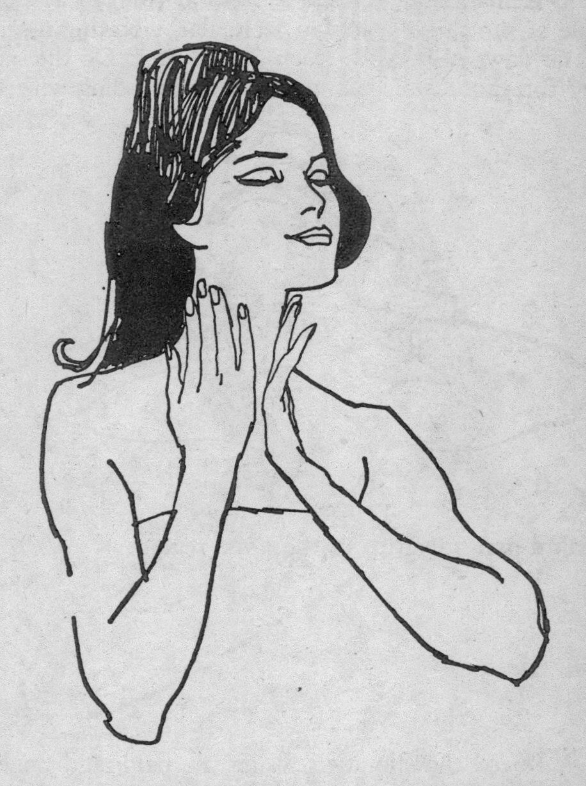

7. Let your head slump forward in a relaxed position as you massage the neck with both hands, making tiny circles with the fingertips.

THE SHOULDERS

8. Still sitting, massage the shoulderblade of each side with the opposite arm. Use a circular movement with the fingertips.

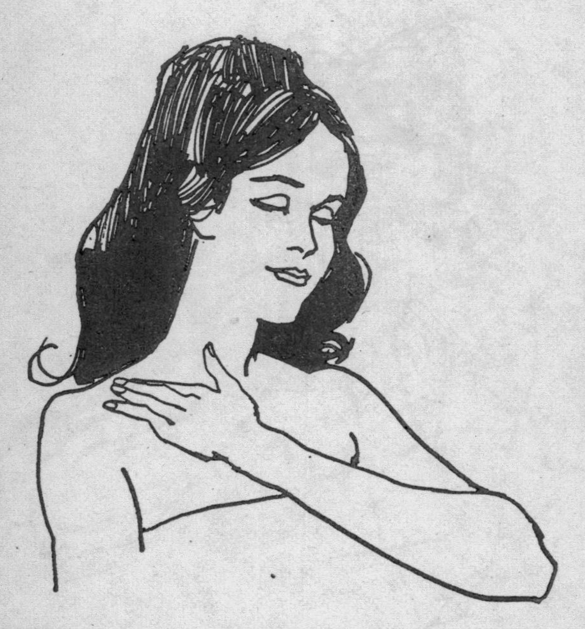

9. Knead the shoulders, using the palm and fingers. Both sides may be done at the same time.

THE ARMS

10. While lying or sitting, work from the wrists to the elbow, and then from the elbow to the shoulder. First knead the muscles in front and back with the palms and the fingertips. The upper arm yields to heavy

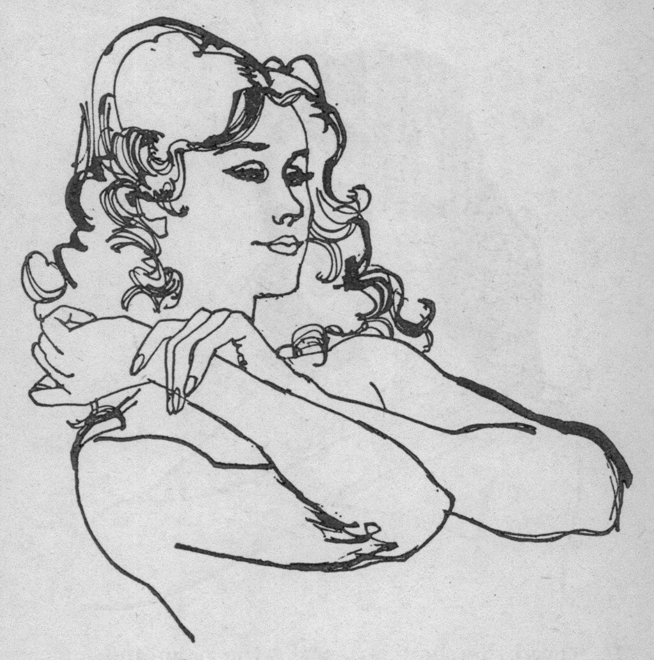

kneading with the palms and the fingertips.

11. Do systematic stroking with the fingertips, making small circular movements.

THE HANDS

12. Work the palms of one hand at a time with the knuckles of the other hand. Bore in, with a rhythmic back-and-forth motion.

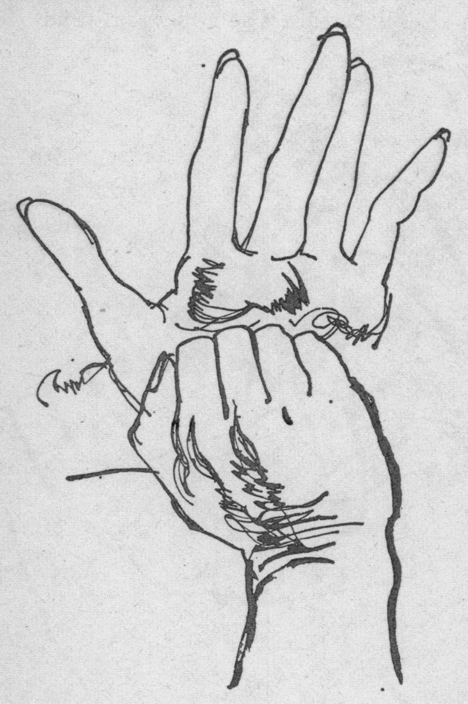

13. Do the same thing, working systematically, with the fingertips or the thumbs.

14. For the front of the hand, using knuckles first, and then fingertips or thumbs, work in the furrows on either side of the ligaments that run from the wrist to the knuckles.

15. Massage the entire front of the hands with the fingertips, making little circular movements.

THE FINGERS

16. Work each finger, one at a time, moving slowly in a corkscrew motion.

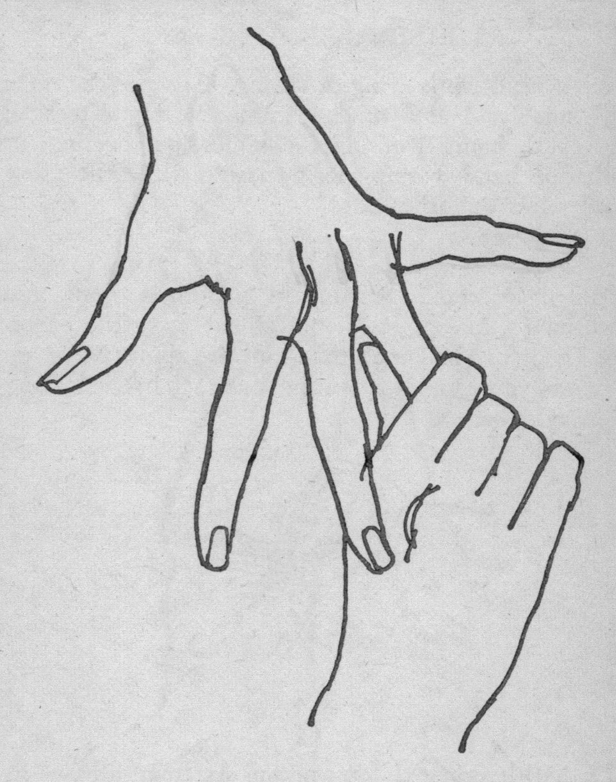

THE CHEST

17. Lie down. Make circular movements with the fingertips, moving systematically over the chest area. Knead with the fingertips.

THE STOMACH

18. Use one palm to rub in a circular motion. Then knead with both hands.

THE SIDES OF THE TORSO

19. Knead while lying or sitting. This may be done with one hand at a time, working the opposite side; with both hands working the same side together; or with one hand working its own side while the other hand works the other side.

THE BACK

20. Sit or stand. Starting at the lower spine, use both hands, make circular movements with the fingertips about one-half inch out from the spine. Move up as far as you can go, repeating this inch-by-inch along the way.

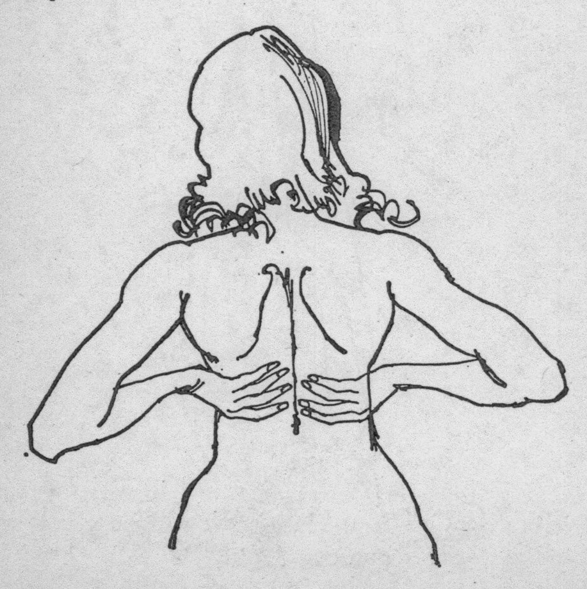

21. The same may be done for the upper back starting at the neck and moving down. Move slowly and systematically; try to press at the side of each vertebra.

THE LEGS

22. Leg strokes may be done either lying down on the floor or on the bed, with feet propped up against the wall. It may also be done sitting up. Many of the strokes in the last chapter may be adapted for self-massage in this position. Strokes are done on one leg at a time.

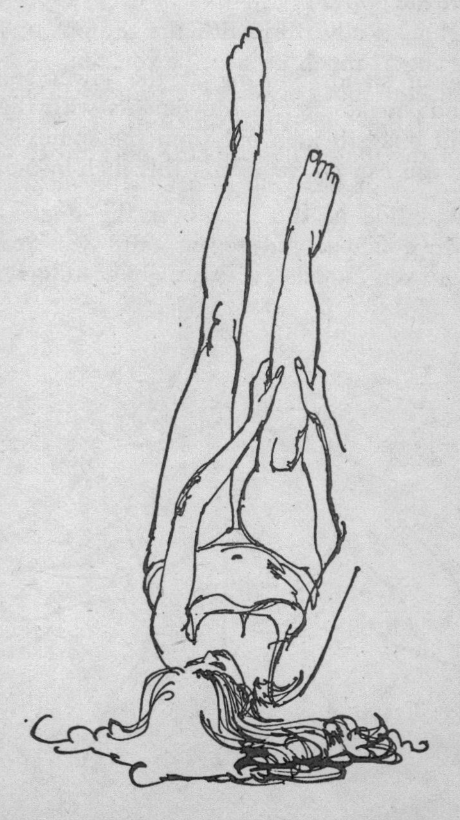

23. Kneading is particularly good here. Use both hands.

24. Pressure may also be applied with the fingertips.

THE BUTTOCKS

25. This must be done lying on the stomach. Knead one side at a time with both hands.

THE FEET

These strokes are best done sitting with the foot resting on the opposite thigh.

26. Systematically work with the thumbs or the fingers, exerting as much pressure as you can.

27. Hold the foot between the palmar surface of the thumbs and the fingertips. Start on the center of the bottom of the foot. Then squeeze outward to the side of the foot, as if breaking a loaf of bread. Move out along the inside of the foot over the fingers underneath. Move down, and repeat until you reach the heel, where you may do some heavy kneading with one hand.

OVERALL

Try slapping the body with both hands—anywhere and everywhere. It's great!

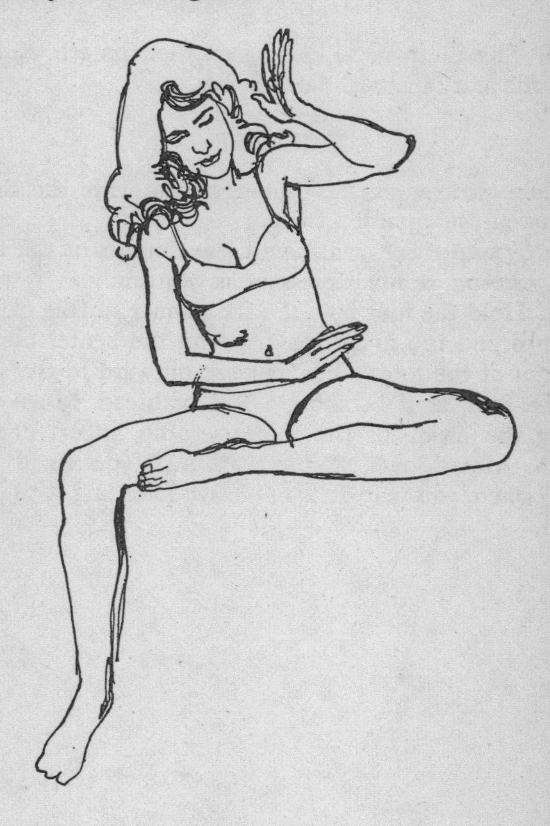

A Bathtub Self-Massage

This is done in a warm, sudsy bath.

THE FACE

1. Any of the self-massage strokes are applicable.

THE LEGS

2. Prop the foot up against the bottom of the tub. Circle the ankle with both hands, thumbs on top. Then stroke up to the knee. Slide back and repeat, kneading the back of the calf muscles with both hands.

3. Shift the hands around and use the fingers to knead the front of the leg.

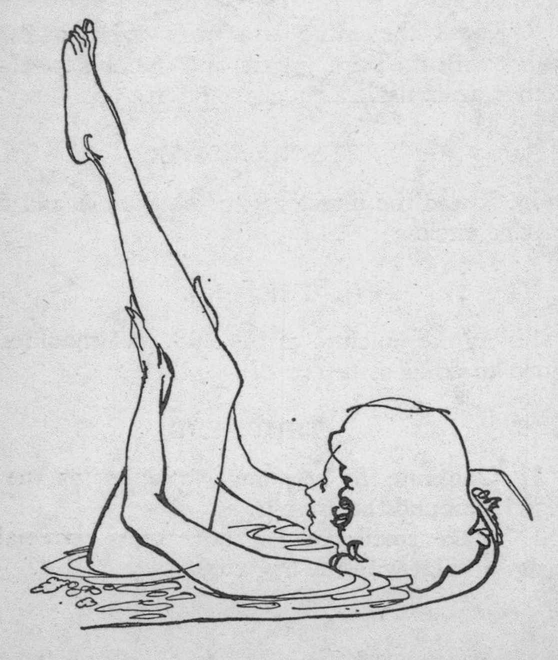

4. Bend the knee. Knead the kneecap on top with fingertips and under the crook of the leg with fingers or thumbs moving in a circular motion.

5. Knead the muscles of the thigh with both hands, working from the knee to the hip.

THE BUTTOCKS

6. Rub your buttocks back and forth against the bottom of the tub.

THE ARMS

7. Work from the wrist to the elbow. Circle the arm at the wrist with the thumb and the fingers. Then knead the muscles.

8. At the elbow, massage with the fingers in a circular motion.

9. Knead the entire arm from wrist to shoulder. Work with the palm, fingers, and thumb kept close together, again using a circular motion.

THE SHOULDERS

10. Knead the muscles with the thumbs and fingers making circles.

THE NECK

11. At the juncture of the neck and shoulder, continue kneading as before.

THE CHEST

12. Continue the kneading movement on the chest muscles around the armpits.

13. Make small circular movements systematically over the chest with the fingertips.

THE STOMACH

14. With both hands, either the whole hand or the fingertips, move in a circular direction, making tiny circles.

Some Devices

There are any number of devices on the market to aid in massage or to do the complete job. A small inventory revealed the following: a foot bath, tub hydrotherapy, heating pads, deep-heat back massage, foot massagers, attachments for the tub to produce a whirlpool bath, and vibrators galore. There are also straps, imported seaweed washclothes, body suits, and vibrating chairs. The consensus among most practitioners is that one's hands are the best tool of all. Whirlpool baths, however, are a useful addition, particularly in some musculoskeletal disorders, and they are often recommended by physicians and physical therapists for athletes, as well as others. Most of the large whirlpool baths are extremely expensive and therefore are found mainly in health clubs and hospitals. Only now are manufacturers beginning to produce some smaller models for the home.

Vibrators can be a great benefit for a self-massage. You don't have to exert as much pressure, and concentration can be better focused. Vibrating chairs are also wonderfully relaxing, although I'm not convinced they can do all that's claimed, and they can be quite expensive. Heating pads are very often recommended by physicians for various joint and muscle disorders, aches, pains, and sprains.

For help in purchasing any of the above items, I suggest you consult a health club, the Department of Physical Medicine and Rehabilitation of your local Veterans Administration hospital, or your private physician, therapist, or masseur.

6

The Orthodox View

Live like a warrior! . . . a warrior takes
responsibility for his acts;
for the most trival of acts.
—don Juan, a seventy-year-old
*Yaqui Indian**

Dr. W. T. Liberson, who is chief of the Department of Physical Medicine and Rehabilitation of the Veterans Administration hospital in Miami, warns that a person with troublesome symptoms should see a physician first before receiving massage therapy. For example, he says, although a pure "tension headache" may be helped by massage, the headaches may be a symptom of a serious disorder. He also rules out general massage for all cardiac patients. The only exception is in the case of cardiac arrest, and for this a cardiac massage must be done immediately. For the most part, I agree with Dr. Liberson's claims. Anyone with severe, repeated headaches should see a good physician, as should someone who is bleeding or in severe pain. But I do think that generally the medical profession tends to be too clannish and parochial in their approach. They can't always see the entire or larger problem. Often someone in another healing art might have a better cure.

* as told to Carlos Castaneda, A Separate Reality, New York, Pocket Books, 1972

A good example of this limited vision is illustrated by the controversy over acupuncture. For years the medical profession in this country and most of the Western world denied the value of acupuncture. Now they are starting to accept the overwhelming evidence that acupuncture can be used successfully to anesthetize the patient as well as to relieve the pain of many disorders. Our own medical profession took a long time to see the merits of acupuncture because they practice allopathic medicine, which is a purely symptomatic approach. They are concerned with applying a counteracting procedure if the body should deviate from the norm: for constipation, they use laxatives; for fever, they attempt to reduce the fever. Acupuncture arises out of a different concept, one which considers the body as a whole and strives to maintain health, not "cure" for particular ailments. In ancient days in China the doctor was paid to keep a patient well, and if the patient got sick, the doctor was penalized, even on occasion beheaded. To people who think in terms of symptoms, as do our own allopathic physicians, sticking needles or applying finger pressure in the thumb and big toe to offset a potential headache makes little sense.

When must we become our own doctors?

How many times have we heard doctors and laymen alike speak of nature being the best healer? Or faith healers talking of miraculous cures? There is a similar element in all of these "cures"—call it autosuggestion or self-hypnosis. This self-healing can be achieved by "listening" to one's own body much as the existential psychologist Rollo May did when he was a child and had tuberculosis. After implicitly following his doctor's orders and resting in bed, he was not getting better. Out of his despair he made the conscious decision to "listen" to his own body. In so doing he became well and gained a new "power." This is a power, I feel, we all have within us; it only needs to be developed. All it takes is gaining a sensitivity to our own body. A small example of this sensitivity can be seen when we have a generalized infection like the flu or a cold, and our body craves certain foods and rejects others. Or by the way we can "feel a cold coming on."

I, for one, feel that all of us must ultimately take responsibility for own bodies. Not that physicians are necessarily wrong, but there are a few decided disadvantages to orthodox Western medicine. First, they treat symptoms primarily, so we have to learn to keep ourselves well. Second, they must become accustomed to nonquestioning acceptance from patients. Overworked, they do not take the time to inform or teach the patient. An extreme example of this is the recent case of a New York doctor who was investigated because of his practice of giving dangerous addicting amphetamines to his patients—some very well-known people—without always telling them what drug they were receiving.

My final advice is to see your physician if you think the symptoms are severe, or if they warrant it. Then, if standard medicine doesn't help, try other methods: chiropractic, osteopathic manipulation, massage, rolfing.

An Interview With A Physiatrist

The member of the medical profession most familiar with massage as part of his everyday practice is the physiatrist, or specialist in physical medicine and rehabilitation. He regularly prescribes massage for his patients, as well as performing all forms of manual medicine, which includes the so-called manipulation and mobilization as well as using modalities such as heat, electricity, and hydrotherapy. Such a specialist is W. T. Liberson, M.D., Ph.D., who, in addition to his duties at the V.A. hospital in Miami, is president of the North American Academy of Manipulative Medicine.

Despite his impressive achievements white-haired Dr. Liberson is almost cherubic and he is as bright-eyed as a boy. In his slow and measured voice, slightly tinged with a European accent, he spoke of many things.

Q: Do you do the massage yourself? I mean, generally, does the physician himself do the massage, or does a physical therapist do it?

A: Manipulation should be done by a physician. The massage may be done by a physical therapist, and usually masseurs [or masseuses] are not prepared to apply therapeutic massage. They usually do a general massage or a massage for a normal individual.

Q: When do you feel a person should have a general body massage?

A: A general body massage has the same indication as general exercise. In other words, a person who would like to have his muscles tonified in general, who wants to have a great deal of autonomic-nervous-system stimulation, might have a generalized massage. People do not realize that skin is a point of origin of a considerable number of reflexes in the autonomic nervous system, which controls articulation in particular and also a great number of cells. Therefore a general massage has a good effect on the peripheral circulation, and may in certain cases lead to a relaxation after the tonic effect wears off. It would be a mistake to consider that this is inoffensive therapy if a person feels that he is not enjoying perfect health.

Q: Do you think that unlicensed or licensed masseurs or masseuses cause damage to people?

A: I don't think so. I went to school here to watch the masseurs, and I understand they are very conscientious and scrupulous people. Unfortunately, this cannot always be said for the general public. The general public feels that the masseur may give them answers that should be the domain of physicians. And the female masseurs [masseuses] are often forced to abandon this occupation . . . after working very hard, because of the continuous demand of their male clients who are convinced that inasmuch as they're masseurs, they have to respond in all possible ways.

Q: As a physiatrist, you use mobilization and manipulation as well as massage. What is that?

A: Imagine a patient sitting in a chair and a doctor taking the patient's head in his hands and trying to turn his hands, let's say, from mid-position to the left. The doctor will try to turn it as much as possible up until the point where he finds resistance. This maneuver is called "mobilization." He can try to give an additional thrust, for which he has to be extremely skilled and very careful, and to do this he must have a knowledge of the condition of that particular patient. With this additional thrust he has an extra movement which ordinarily is not under voluntary control of the patient. Then this mobilization becomes a "manipulation." And it is usually associated with a "pop." This could be very dangerous, and it should be done by a physician.

Q: What sort of disorders are usually treated by manual medicine, outside of disorders of the musculoskeletal system, which I understand are the most commonly treated?

A: The whole gamut of disorders which affect the

joints, the ligaments, the tendons, the muscles, and the nervous system.

Q: Do you think the typical tired executive or housewife, or person who has to stand on his feet all day long and feels very tense, is a good candidate for general body massage?

A: If you are asking me whether a physician after examining a patient and arriving at the conclusion that there is nothing wrong except an ordinary fatigue—yes, I think this is possible. But first he has to be sure that there is no hidden disease and that a patient is not a cardiac patient.

Q: Could massage actually hurt a cardiac patient?

A: Oh, yes.

Q: How so? If it improves the circulation, I would think it would help a cardiac patient.

A: Massage improves the peripheral circulation of the skin. Whenever you have more blood in a certain area of the body, you take some blood from some other part of the body. Therefore, when you do this in a cardiac patient you may reduce the amount of blood which is necessary in the coronary arteries or the arteries of the brain; I would not recommend this in a cardiac patient.

Q: Why can't you massage just the chest area—the heart—in a cardiac patient?

A: At the present time there is a procedure which is life-saving—having a deep massage over the cardiac area in a patient who has a cardiac arrest. A lay person can be trained to do this. It is a life-saving sort of massage, and it is done only when there is a cardiac arrest.

How To Save A Life:
The Principles of Cardiac Massage

> If you are an American, there is a greater than 50% chance that you will die from a circulatory disease.
> If you are an adult male, or a female approaching the menopause, you probably already have a disease of the arteries to your heart or other vital organs.
> Almost everyone in the U.S. and in most of the industrialized countries of the world today either has a disease of the heart or blood vessels or has a member of the immediate family or close friend with such a disorder.

These dramatic statements were made by Lawrence E. Lamb, M.D., in *Your Heart and How to Live with It*, published in 1969. Because heart disease is so prevalent, sooner or later almost everyone is confronted with the problem of what to do about a person who has lost consciousness either from a simple faint or because of a heart attack. Prompt assistance is needed at such times. The following rules tell when and how to perform a cardiac massage.

If someone suddenly collapses, first find out if the person is still breathing. If breathing has stopped, do mouth-to-mouth resuscitation as follows: (1) Place a pillow under the victim's shoulder if possible; (2) bend the head back to clear the passage to the lungs; (3) place one hand in back of the victim's neck; (4) pinch off the nostrils with the other hand; (5) seal your lips around the victim's open mouth to shut off loss of air; (6) blow air forcibly into the open mouth, removing your mouth to inhale and to allow air to exhale from the victim's mouth. Repeat and maintain a regular rhythm of inhaling and exhaling. This can be continued by someone else as you do the following:

find out if the person has a pulse or not. Feel the wrist above the thumb, the temple just in front of the ear, the neck just below the jaw, and the chest just below the left breast. If you can feel no pulse, assume that circulation has stopped. Try to start the heart beating again by striking a sharp blow with your fist just to the left of the breastbone (sternum) and below the nipple. If the heart has not started, stroke the chest again. If the above procedure fails to start the heart, do a cardiac massage as follows:

1. Get down on knees, facing the victim.
2. Place the heel of one hand directly on the lower part of the sternum (breastbone) just above the pit of the stomach. The hand should not be over the stomach.
3. Place your other hand over it to reinforce it, and keeping the elbows straight, rise up and then apply a downward pressure directly upon the sternum. The effective pressure in an adult is about seventy pounds, or enough to push the sternum down toward the backbone about two inches. This movement squeezes the blood out of the heart into the arteries.
4. Release your pressure to allow the sternum to snap back into place. During this period the heart refills with blood.
5. This procedure should be repeated, as if replacing the normal beating of the heart. It is done about sixty times a minute, or one downward stroke per second.

If there is not someone else present to do the mouth-to-mouth breathing, stop about every twenty seconds, close off the nostrils, and exhale three times into the lungs of the victim.

If the heartbeat returns and respiration remains normal, the victim should be left lying comfortably until medical assistance can be obtained.

In the case of children, the fingers of each hand can be wrapped around the child's back, with thumbs on the middle of the sternum and the hands placed roughly mid-chest. Pressure is applied with the thumbs, while still attempting to provide a movement of about two inches. This should require less pressure in an infant.

A Physical Therapist Answers Some Questions

Robert Panzenbeck is a licensed physical therapist in private practice in New York City, with a master's degree in physical therapy. He has a large and busy professional practice. All of his patients are referred by various physicians with specific instructions as to treatment, in keeping with the law of New York State. Mr. Panzenbeck generally expressed the view that too few physicians or physical therapists know the benefits of massage, and they don't use it often enough because "it's old, and you have to get your hands dirty." He, on the other hand, uses it in about ninety-five percent of the patients who are sent to him. He feels also that physical therapists and physicians are not being taught enough in the schools about the use of massage. Certain areas of the body are neglected, he feels, insofar as massage is concerned—the feet, for example, and the elbows, and possibly the face.

Q: I understand all physical therapists use exercise and "modalities" in addition to massage. What is that?
A: Either deep heat or whirlpool, or I instruct my patients to use ice at home.

Q: Do you use heat with the massage?
A: Yes, I use both together.

Q: For what kind of conditions?
A: Low back strain, tightness of the neck ... a lot of different conditions.

Q: Do you get many patients with arthritic conditions?

A: Yes. I particularly get a lot of patients with arthritis of the back or spine.

Q: Do you ever do a general body massage?

A: I mostly massage parts. It depends on the doctor's orders. One time a doctor sent a lot of former drug addicts to me for general massage. I became angered and told the doctor that I was not accustomed to so much general-massage work. He told me something I will always remember, that "massage is to physical therapy what a hypodermic is to a doctor."

Q: Do you find the work rewarding?

A: Yes, I find it very rewarding. It is also rewarding financially. I would like to see many more people taking up this field, particularly going into private practice. One of my teachers, at the Hospital for Special Surgery in New York, told us to use our hands, that it is the greatest tool we have with a patient. And patients know once you lay your hands on them whether or not you know what you're doing.

On Osteopathy

It wasn't too long ago that osteopaths were excluded from any professional commerce with the orthodox medical community (as represented by the American Medical Association), much as the chiropractor, who is still considered an enemy by many in the Establishment.* Now, however, osteopaths can call themselves

*Chiropractic is an entire system of drugless treatment based on the principle that a person's health is determined largely by his nervous system and that interference with this system impairs a person's normal functioning and lowers the resistance to disease. Chiropractors treat primarily by manual manipulation of part of the body, especially the spinal column. This is a very sophisticated

doctors and prescribe medication much as any physician. They are generally a part of the orthodoxy, and in some small communities—particularly in the Midwest—often the only doctor in the community is an osteopath and the only hospital is an osteopathic hospital. What distinguishes osteopaths from other practitioners is their method of manipulation, which evolved from the work of a former country doctor, Andrew Taylor Still. His explanation of disease was "the rule of the artery: wherever blood is circulating normally, disease cannot develop because our blood is capable of manufacturing all the necessary substance to maintain natural immunity against disease." He felt the cause of all diseases to be a partial or complete failure of the nerves " . . . to properly conduct the fluids of life." By manipulation he tried to restore the body's structural integrity by getting the nervous system to function once more. Dr. Still himself distrusted massage, but many osteopaths today prescribe it in addition to other treatment. When you read the next chapter, on acupuncture, you may notice the similarity between Dr. Still's theory and the theory of Oriental medicine as used in acupuncture. A practitioner of Oriental medi-

---

and skilled method, and they deny it has much, if anything, to do with massage. They also use measures such as light and heat therapy, and they prescribe diet, exercise, and rest. They use X rays for diagnosis. Chiropractic has long been rejected in this country in orthodox medical circles, although there are now about 16,000 practicing chiropractors throughout the United States. The British Medical Association now recognizes chiropractic manipulation as a part of its medicine, and Dr. James Cyriax, a leading British orthopedist, has performed or prescribed manipulation for 40,000 patients, particularly for backaches. I believe it is well worth investigating. For more information, write the National College of Chiropractic, 220 East Roosevelt Road, Lombard (Chicago), Illinois 60148; or New York State Chiropractic Association, 45 John Street, New York, New York 10038; or the chiropractic association in your state.

cine, Dr. Zerinsky, claims that "for years osteopaths have been practicing acupuncture and they don't know it."

An Interview With Two Osteopaths

The Leroy Hospital is the only osteopathic hospital in Manhattan. It has the facilities of a regular hospital, only osteopathic manipulations are also performed. There is also a full-time physical therapist on staff to do massage when doctors prescribe it. I interviewed the acting dean of their Postgraduate Institute, which is located at the hospital. He is William D. Miller, D.O. I also interviewed William O. Kingsbury, D.O., professor of osteopathic principles and practice.

Q: Dr. Miller, when would you encourage a person to see an osteopath?

M: We are the general practitioners. The family physicians. I find D.O.'s are the best physicians all around. Osteopaths have done a lot for me personally. I started in osteopathy because as a child I kept getting colds. My mother sent me to an osteopath, and after he treated me I didn't catch colds. I started to put on weight. The whole neighborhood then went to him. We believe in results.

Q: Most people I know would consider osteopathy something to be used mostly for disease of the joints or muscles. Is this true?

M: Why do you think we have a hospital? It is for patients who need acute medical care. We have a complete service. We have osteopathic surgeons, osteopathic psychiatrists, and so forth. In the Midwest, where osteopathy started, many smaller communities have only an osteopathic hospital or physician. When an osteopath graduates from school, he's a physician. There are only two types of physicians in the United States today. There are the allopathic physicians and the osteopaths. But we are the only two. Chiropractors are not physicians; physiotherapists are not. Only we. We give complete health care.

Q: Can you give me an example of a case in which pure osteopathy can be applied?

M: We're doing such a study right now. Chronic obstructed pulmonary diseases, such as asthma, bronchitis, and emphysema. Conventional therapy hasn't been very successful in these conditions.

K: We also saved—and this was before 1938, before the days of antibiotics and sulfa—the lives of a great many people with influenza and pneumonia through osteopathic manipulative treatment. The osteopathic profession gained strength at that time by successfully treating many people who were given up for dead by the medical profession.

M: Remember, there was no medicine—rather, specifics—then for these diseases. The number-one killers at that time were the infectious diseases. The osteopathic physicians would treat their patients manipulatively, and they had a much lower mortality rate than other physicians.

Q: Dr. Kingsbury, do you prescribe massage often?

K: I encourage my patients when they ask about massage. I say, "If you have a well-qualified masseur and you get a benefit from it, I certainly would go ahead and have it." Mostly these are people seeking relaxation, and perhaps having a problem coping with daily life. I feel massage can offer ancillary benefit in certain patients. Many people that I know and come in contact with have massage two or three times a week.

Massage In Dentistry

All dentists recommend regular massage of the gums as part of good dental prophylaxis. Dr. Raymond Levao, who practices in New York, outlined his recommendations.

1. Use a soft-bristled brush. At first Dr. Levao urged his patients to use the Oral B brush, but now he says there are others like it on the market, such as the Butler brush. The important feature is that the brush be soft and malleable and the bristles fit nicely to the contours of the mouth. When rubbed against the gums, the brush serves to stimulate the formation of a dense mucosa. This helps normal tissues get the proper stimulation; the foods we eat are usually cooked and soft, and consequently our gums don't get enough stimulation and thus break down and easily become infiltrated by bacteria.

To massage with this brush, first relax your mouth. Do not attempt to smile or posture as you insert the toothbrush. Starting at the back, place the brush perpendicular to the gums and teeth. Remain in this position for about fifteen seconds, applying pressure so the bristles spread out, and move in a circular direction without lifting the toothbrush from the area. Now move to a position about one-fourth inch closer to the center of the mouth. Repeat. Continue on the top and bottom and then do the same thing for the back of the teeth. Take your time and do it thoroughly and systematically. At first, time yourself so you take a full three minutes by the clock. Never tense your mouth as you do it or try to open your mouth, for you will miss areas that way.

2. Massage with a rubber tip. The Py-co-pay toothbrush has a rubber tip at its end. This is recommended

to be used for massage between the crevices of the teeth. It is good to do on a daily basis or with certain disorders such as trench mouth, as it stimulates the tissues between the teeth, which are normally soft and delicate and are never exposed to rubbing.

3. The Water Pic. Dr. Levao says that the intermittent flow of water causes a massagelike action on the tissues as it compresses and relaxes the tissue and increases the circulation to the parts.

7

The Orient—Here And There

I have heard that in ancient times the people lived to be over a hundred years, and yet they remained active and did not become decrepit in their activities. But nowadays people only reach half of that age and yet become decrepit and failing.

*Is it that mankind is becoming negligent of the laws of nature? In ancient times those people who understood the Tao, patterned themselves upon the Yin and the Yang . . . .**

Legend has it that an ancient Chinese warlord was pierced by an arrow during a fight, and an illness from which he had been suffering suddenly disappeared; and thus acupuncture began. People also noticed that when they got splinters in their feet in certain places, certain organs responded. This is essentially the way in which Chinese medicine evolved—as in our own Western medicine, out of observation.

Although the science of Oriental medicine dates back some five thousand years, it was only introduced to the Western World in about 1927 when Soulié de Morand, the French consul serving in China, reported on acupuncture. The Jesuit missionaries and French traders had made observations earlier, but they did not publish their experiences. After Monsieur de Morand's report, acupuncture began to gather some momentum in France and attracted some members of the healing arts, particularly among homeopaths—believers in the principle of *Simila similibus curentur*, "Let like be treated by like." (Homeopathy, by the way, is the con-

* The Yellow Emperor's *Nei Jing*, classic of internal medicine

cept upon which the principle of immunization is based.) Acupuncture later gathered disciples in England. But it has been only within the past few years that people in high places in the United States have come to regard it as tenable. The well-known physician, Walter Tkach, M.D., reported that on his tour of China he had seen acupuncture at work, and it so impressed him that he says he would not hesitate to receive anesthesia by acupuncture himself.

Some evidence that acupuncture works. That the "life force" operates through predetermined meridians is a concept that has been difficult for Westerners to accept. This is surprising, because we accept the existence of energies of gravity and the moon—forces we cannot see. We do use electrocardiography (measurements of the heart), electromyography (which measures electrical potential of muscles), and electroencephalography (a measurement of brain waves), and we accept that these are measurements of some kind of electrical potential of various parts and organs of the body. So why should it be so hard to accept acupuncture?

As early as the nineteenth century, a German doctor, knowing nothing of acupuncture, discovered sensitive skin points. Later, when these points were compared with those on Chinese acupuncture charts, more than three-quarters of them coincided. At about that time the English neurologist Henry Head verified that certain zones on the skin were hypersensitive to pressure if a diseased organ was connected by nerves to the region.

A Russian physiologist did studies measuring the electrical potential of the skin at the classical acupuncture points. He used X rays, encephalography, and electrocardiography, and the results verified the basic claims of acupuncturists. Experiments to date have shown that electrical conductivity at some 690 points on the skin, relating to acupuncture points, is much higher than for the rest of the skin.

Confirmation of a more practical kind came about in the 1950's when a doctor in Korea developed an electrical machine which, when passed over the surface of the skin, would react at certain points, which coincided with those on the old Chinese charts. The machine gave an impetus to the practice of acupuncture in the West, and anybody could treat patients with the help of a few charts, using the "magic eye" of the electroacupuncture machine.

The basic theory. The Oriental system of medicine includes not only what Westerners know as acupuncture —from *acus*, "needles" and *punctura*, "to pierce"—but the Chinese medical system, which they call "needle and burning," also includes moxibustion (healing with heat and fire), herbal treatment, breathing therapy, and massage. Because China is an immense country which encompasses many different climates, and in ancient times included many "alien races," the folk medicine differed from region to region, and each area had its own system of treatment. Medicinal herbs were used in one area, exercise and baths in another, and massage in still another. What serves to unify the system comes out of Taoist belief—that man is an integral part of a live universe, and harmony is a basic principle of the world order.

Essentially, they believe that in a normal individual there is a continuous flow of energy. This energy, or *Qi*, flows through certain channels, called meridians. At various points on these fourteen meridians, there are certain peculiarly sensitive areas, the so-called acupuncture points. If needles or pressure is applied at these points, it will influence an organ related to the meridian on which the point lies. The theory is that if any part of the body is suffering from a disorder, the flow in the meridian which serves that organ or part will diminish. This disturbs the integrity of the body and causes illness. Therefore, by pricking at a number of carefully selected points, or pressing with the fingers at these points, the skilled practitioner can reestablish the normal circulation of energy and restore a person to health, provided the tissues have not yet been destroyed.

The body is considered a microcosm of the universe. There is a constant struggle in the human organism, just as in nature, between opposing and unifying forces; and good and bad health are determined by fluctuations between poles—yin and yang. This concept is difficult for a Westerner to comprehend, and as a woman I find it somewhat offensive, in that the yin is classified as weakness, darkness, the negative—the feminine; while yang is classified as strength, lightness, the positive—the masculine. Everything in the universe, including every organ in the human body, is classified according to yin and yang. The solid organs, such as the liver, lungs, and heart, are yin; and the hollow organs, such as the intestines and stomach, are yang.

Diagnosis according to this system is highly complex. As it is a system of maintaining health rather than treating symptoms, the person is looked upon as a whole. His color, speech, and movement are studied. The many different pulses are touched—this is a very refined art which takes years to develop. Some Oriental practitioners never totally develop the skill to its finest potential, for this requires learning how to detect minute variations in the many pulses of the body. In China, Dr. Zerinsky claims, there are three types of physician: one who can read the body mentally making note of signs, which can aid him in treating a person to prevent him from getting ill; the second type of physician needs symptoms; and the third is the "master," who can move energy through the body, using the mind alone.

An Interview With a Western Practitioner of the Oriental Method

Dr. Sidney Zerinsky, a modest-looking man with exquisitely smooth, beautifully constructed white hands, is principal of the Swedish Institute for Massage in New York City. He is a licensed physical therapist, with his doctorate in naturopathic medicine. In addition to running the Institute, he is in private practice and is a student of Oriental medicine.

Q: Dr. Zerinsky, what would you say is the success rate of acupuncture?

A: Acupuncture doesn't help everyone; in about six or seven cases out of ten it works. No form of Chinese medicine can change tissue structure, so if there's tissue damage, it can't be helped. But acupuncture can relieve pain. I think it's the same as with any practitioner: they help you twenty-five percent; you help yourself seventy-five percent.

Q: What about Oriental massage?

A: It's good if the practitioner works in these same acupuncture areas. It won't last too long. It only temporarily balances the meridians' vital force or energy.

Q: In what conditions would you say the Oriental system of massage works best?

A: Musculoskeletal problems—sprains, strains, back ailments, sciatica. Headaches. Stomach problems. I don't advise it for someone with arthritis of the spine.

Q: In what conditions would you recommend a general body massage?

A: Essentially the same ones I mentioned before. It is also very good for convalescence—for elderly people and for people that have a disease that's incapacitated them for a long time, and so they must be bedridden. Massage is also very helpful for various forms of paralysis.

Q: Where does Swedish massage differ from Oriental massage?

A: Basically all massage movements developed out of the Chinese techniques, which consist of about sixty-eight different movements. If you want to translate the Chinese system of massage in modern terms, it would be "push-and-pull" movements. There are many variations of these, and the Swedish system consists of five variations of them—stroking, kneading, friction, vibration, and percussion.

Q: Why do you think they chose those particular five?

A: Massage was introduced to Western civilization when the Portuguese and the Italian Marco Polo went to China. They reported on their observations. And the massage movements that were used finally were probably the ones that seemed the most logical in the thinking of Western man.

Q: How do you make a diagnosis?

A: Diagnosis is a term used in Western medicine. I use the Oriental system, which is far better. We look at the body in many ways—the pulse, the color, the manner in which a person speaks. We look at attitudes as well as the physical complaint. Learning to read the pulses is very difficult; it takes at least fifteen years of study. I'm still studying it.

Q: This is called the Swedish Institute for Massage,

and yet you have pictures of acupuncture points on the wall, and you yourself practice Oriental methods. Do you also teach the Oriental method of massage here?

A: It's against the law now.*

Q: Do you think things will change?

A: Not at all. Not while the AMA is as strong as it is. Right now acupuncture is also illegal.

Q: Can you give me a few examples of how finger pressure at acupuncture points works?

A: I'll give you a few simple examples—some that you can do yourself without getting into trouble. Follow the instructions implicitly, because if you work too long in an area where there is a problem, it could cause a paralysis. This doesn't work on everyone, so do at least three treatments, a maximum of six. If it doesn't help, don't do it anymore.

For "freeing the spirit" within the body, apply pressure at the associated kidney point. This kidney point is located at the palmar surface of both feet, in the middle of the sole between the third and fourth toes. If a person feels listless, dull, lacking in energy, or feels there is something holding him or her back all the time, pressure here can relieve this.

For the stomach and large colon, apply rotary pressure at a forty-five-degree angle in the webbing of the hand between the thumb and forefinger. Do no more than three minutes on each hand. Do about four times a day.

For colds, sinuses, and head congestion, take the

* Presently, according to New York State law, only M.D.s may practice acupuncture. The Chinese "masters," not generally licensed M.D.s, may not practice in New York. In some states they may practice only when supervised by an M.D. The law is in flux, and varies from state to state. Ironically, acupuncture in New York had been practiced in Chinatown for more than one hundred years before this current law came into effect.

thumb and forefinger with your other hand and squeeze the two together hard. Do three minutes on each hand, four times a day.

For ear trouble and hearing problems, take the third and fourth fingers of the side affected. Apply pressure on top of the nail for three minutes on each finger alternately. Do three or four times a day.

For the eyes, exert pressure underneath the second and third toe where the toe meets the sole of the foot, working on the foot that is on the same side as the troubled eye. Press in each spot about three minutes.

People who practice yoga and feel that their body and mind are "separated" can find that pressure at *the psychic point* will unify them. Pressure here may also help develop a psychic state. The point is just below the shoulder level, on the upper arm at the head of the humerus.

For menstrual difficulties, exert pressure with a finger or thumb on the upper back near the shoulder on the point illustrated, on either side of the spine between the fourth and fifth thoracic vertebrae. Don't press more than three minutes.

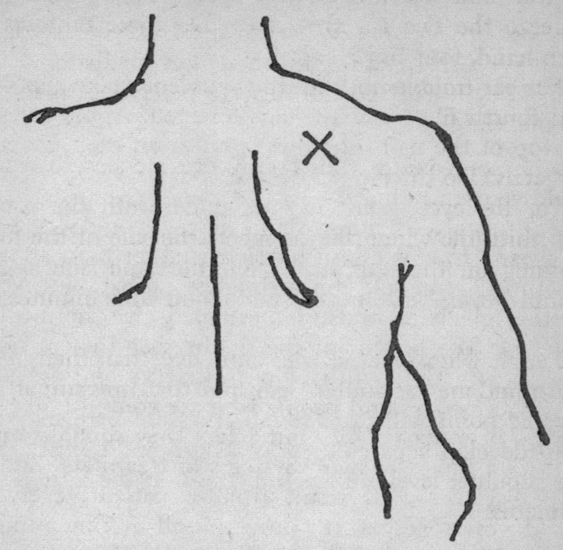

For frontal headache, place thumb in the roof of the mouth and press for five minutes. Do three or four times a day.

To make a relaxing *eye pack,* use bamboo shoots. Wash well and put in cold water. Place the bamboo shoots on eyelids.

Q: Thank you, Dr. Zerinsky. I have just a few more questions to ask you. What do most of your students at the Swedish Institute do when they graduate?

A: They usually go into private practice as masseurs and masseuses.

Q: If someone in your family became sick to whom would you send him?

A: Probably, as things stand now, I would first send the person to a Western physician rather than an acupuncturist. I, myself, am a drugless practitioner, yet I feel that medicine is also important. I give the medical profession the benefit of the doubt that they're really interested in the health of our citizenry and are worried about quacks and people who are going to take advantage of other people. But I feel they should understand that there are many systems of treatment, and to get a better overall result from a patient, everyone should work together. It's proven itself in China today, where Chinese traditional medicine and Western modernized medicine are harmoniously working together and getting very good results for the patient. We in the West have divided the body from the mind, and so we treat only the physical symptoms.

Some Disorders Treated by the Japanese Method

Essentially, the Japanese method is a combination of ancient Chinese massage and Western methods. I have chosen some common disorders for which the treatment is relatively simple. As I mentioned before, if symptoms are severe or persistent, see a physician.

For headache, first wrap a towel around the subject's head and secure it at the base of the neck. This is done with the subject sitting in a relaxed position. Follow the diagram and apply pressure in small circular motions at each point for from three to five minutes. Using the thumbs of both hands, lightly massage points 1 through 7 on either side of the head. Slowly. Do points 8 through 10, around the ears, using the palms. Continue on to point 11, again using the fingertips. If headaches are severe, massage points 12 and 13, under the ear and on the neck. Repeat. The treatment has a greater chance of effectiveness if points 14 through 16 on the body are also done.

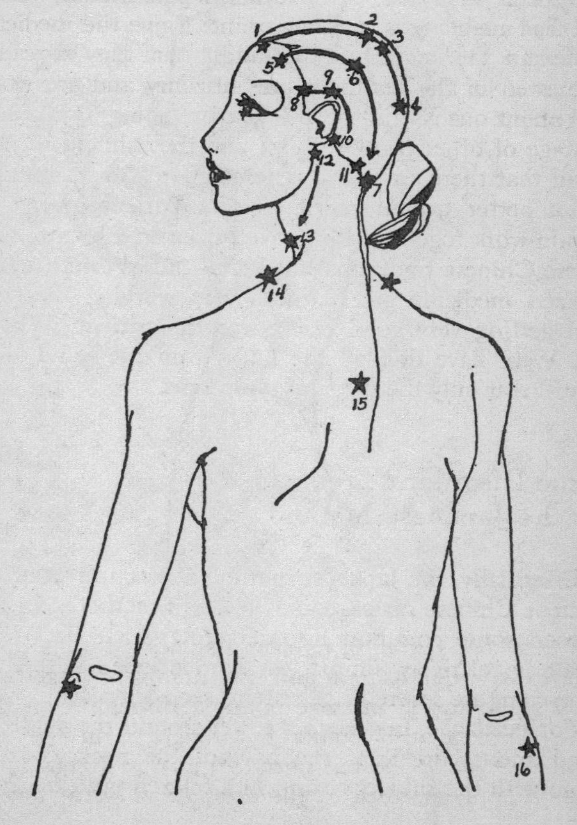

For toothache, the treatment may be done by the subject on herself or himself. Following the diagram, for pain in the teeth of the upper jaw, press or massage point 1 under each eye. Use thumbs (applied from the back to the front) on points 2 and 3. For pain of the teeth in the lower jaw, use pressure near the nose on point 4 and below the mouth on point 5.

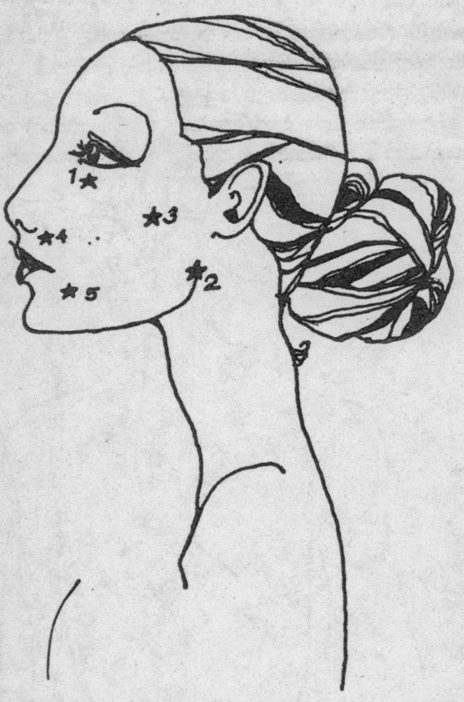

For stomach cramps, Subject assumes a supine position. Follow the diagram and use thumbs or fingertips. During the attack, massage points 1 through 4 on the back. Massage also points 5 through 8 on the abdomen. Seven is located next to the ribs. It may also help to apply warmth to the area, using warm towels or heating pads. Try rubbing both hands together to bring up a warmth, and gently stroke the area. After the attack has subsided, with the subject lying on his or her back, apply pressure with the thumbs, palms, or forefingers to point 9 above each kneecap and 10 on the sides of the calves of the legs.

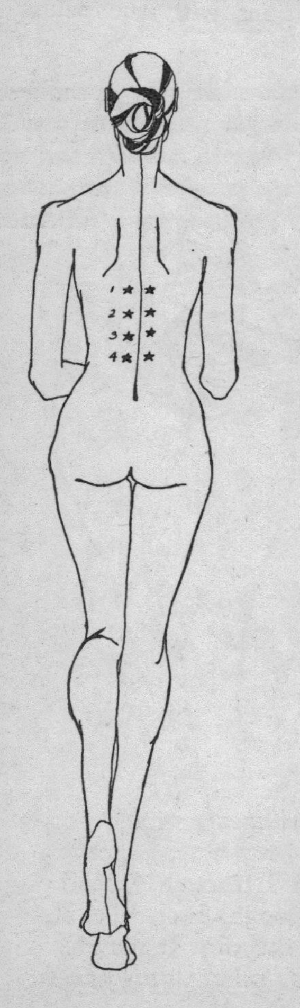

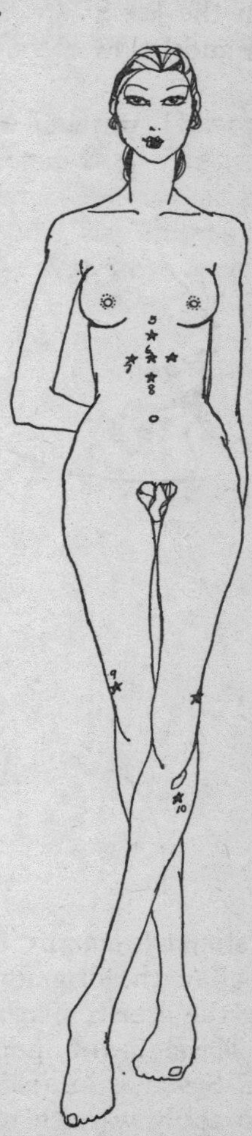

For backache, apply warmth, using a heating pad or warm towels, first to the back, then to the stomach. Do this for about one-half hour. Next, place one hand on top of the other, and using the palm of one hand, massage in the direction shown in the diagram, first, in the direction of A, then B and C, on the subject's back. Make small circular motions with the palms.

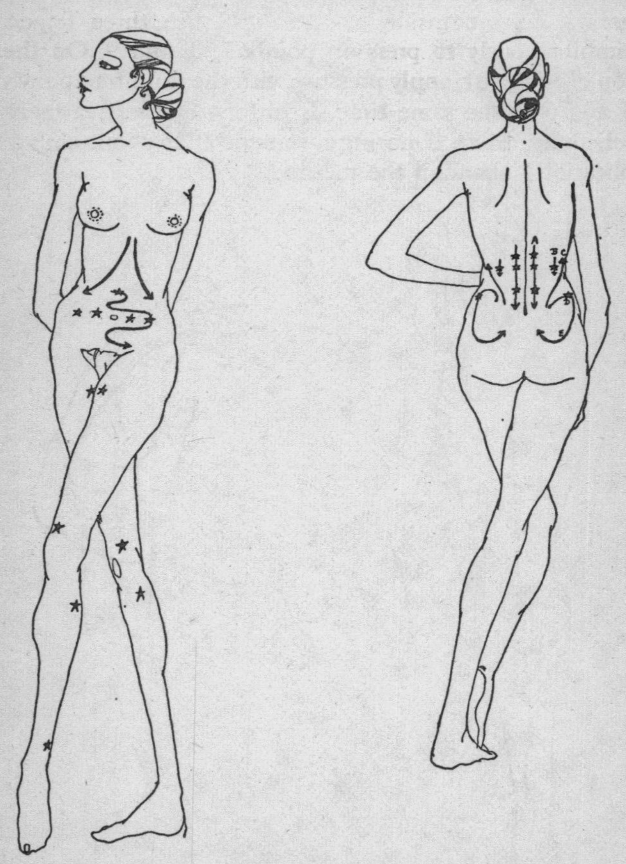

Using the thumbs, apply pressure at area D. Massage the buttocks—E—with the palms of both hands in a circular direction. On the subject's front, massage and use finger pressure following the direction shown. Warm baths can also aid in reducing pain.

For rheumatism, the application of warmth helps the affected joints. Apply pressure at the points in the diagram. On the inside of the wrist, use three fingers simultaneously to press on points 7, 8, and 9. On the top of the wrist, apply pressure with the thumb to points 5 and 6 at the same time. If, in any of the treatment schedules, there is no improvement after about six applications, abandon the method.

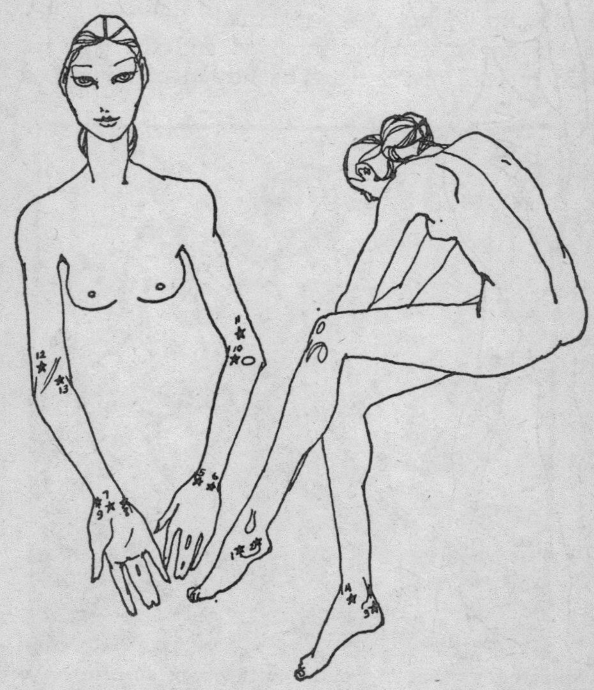

The Ancient Art of "Cupping"

For more than two thousand years Chinese physicians have used cups made out of animal horns, bamboo tubes, burned clay, or glass. Other ancient people performed a similar technique by sucking in with the mouth. Though not strictly classified as a massage technique, cupping is sometimes used as an accompaniment to massage. In the modern method we mix medicinal herbs with oil or alcohol in an ordinary glass tumbler of about two or three inches in diameter. Then we take cotton or paper and soak it briefly. A match is applied to the material, and with this we warm the mixture. When the glass starts to get extremely hot, the burning material is removed and the glass is allowed to cool just a bit. The heated cupping glass is

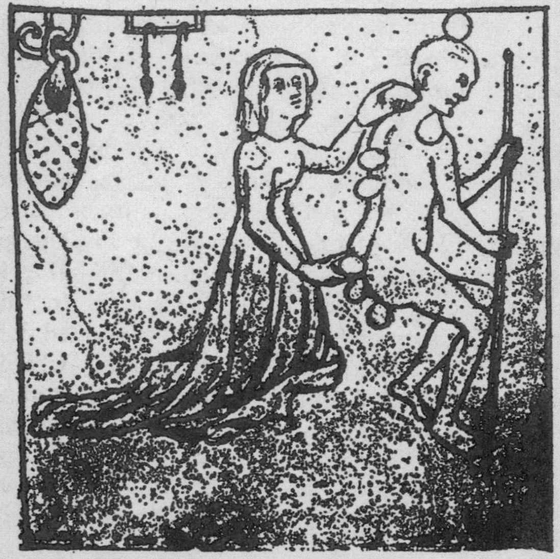

Miniature drawing of woman putting cups on man, 1350. Woodcut. *(Courtesy The Bettman Archive, New York.)*

then placed, edge down, on the part of the body to be treated, and left for ten to fifteen minutes. The flesh will rise quite dramatically into the cup. To remove, tip the cup on its side.

Cupping has been used in the treatment of colds and rheumatic ailments, abdominal pains, and headaches. It should never be used for skin diseases, abscesses, and infectious diseases of any kind, or on the abdomen of pregnant women.

Some Related Western Therapies: Zone Therapy, Dō-in, and Polarity Therapy

Have you ever stopped an impending sneeze by pressing under your nose with your forefinger? Or put your warm hands on your stomach when it hurt? Do you remember as a child when your mother stopped a nosebleed by pressing some ice against the back of your neck? These are folk remedies that utilize principles that are a part of a system of treatment called zone therapy, or reflexology. When someone clenches his hands or grits his teeth to stop pain, or caresses a bumped shin, the reflexologist might say the person was stopping the transmission of nerve impulses in the "zone" related to the affected body part. In this system, as in acupuncture, the body is divided longitudinally into "zones." Unlike acupuncture, which uses fourteen meridians, zone therapy utilizes ten zones, each ending at the toes. There are five to each side of the body, and they begin in the fingers and run up the hands and arms, over the face and head, and down the front and back of the body, ending in the feet and toes.

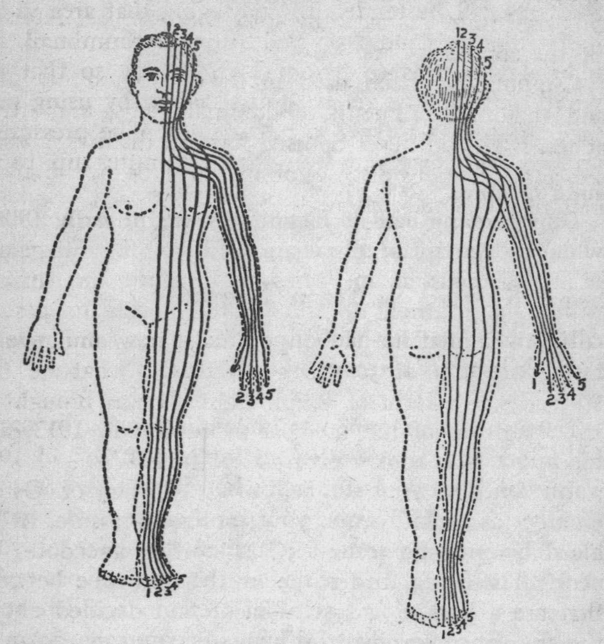

(left) Diagram of Posterior Zones on one side of the body. Both right and left sides of the body are the same. Each numbered line represents the center of its respective zone on the posterior part of the body. *(From Wm. H. Fitzgerald, 1917.)* (right) Diagram of Anterior Zones on one side of the body. Both right and left sides of the body are the same. Each numbered line represents the center of its respective zone on the anterior part of the body. *(From Wm. H. Fitzgerald, 1917.)*

Eunice D. Ingham, the foremost living practitioner of zone therapy, claims that if every cell in the body contracts and relaxes as nature intends, we would have perfect health and perfect feet. However, if congestion should take place in any part of the body, the "nerve reflex area" to that particular organ, which is located in the feet, will be tender. By massaging that area in the foot with the thumb or well-trimmed thumbnail, the reflexologist aims to "ground" the body so that the nerve reflexes flow freely. This is done by using pressure equivalent to two to ten pounds. The pressure is applied for anywhere from three minutes up to an hour or more.

Zone therapy had its beginnings in the early 1900's, when an American physician, William H. Fitzgerald, M.D., studied at an Oriental institute in Austria. When he returned to the United States, he ecstatically proclaimed he had discovered a new and revolutionary system of treatment. Actually, what he had studied was a form of acupuncture. It was brought to the attention of the medical profession in 1913, and his now classic book was published in 1917.

Earlier, Dr. Andrew Still, the "Father of Osteopathy," had noted the effect of applied pressure. In his autobiography he related an interesting anecdote. He wanted to swing, and so he hung some rope between two trees, but he had a headache and decided not to use it. For some odd reason, he let the rope down to about eight inches from the ground, and, lying on the ground, he used the rope as a "swinging pillow." He lay there stretched out on his back with his neck across the rope and soon fell asleep. When he awoke, his headache was gone. From that time on, he roped his neck whenever he had a headache. He claims by doing this he ". . . had suspended the action of the great occipital nerves, and given harmony to the flow of arterial blood to and through the veins, and ease was the effect." Whatever the actual process involved, some disorders do seem to respond to what sound like folk remedies and these remedies are often similar to what has been systematized into the practice of zone therapy. I must confess I haven't tried them myself with any regularity, but I am giving a few examples that a person may apply on himself or a friend without much difficulty. The more complicated methods, some using probes or needles, I leave to the medical or dental profession; zone therapy has had some apparent success, particularly in dentistry, as an anesthesia. The following are some simple procedures you might try. I make no guarantees.

For headache, the treatment is basically the same as Dr. Zerinsky's acupuncture remedy. First wash the hands. Then insert two fingers in the subject's mouth. For self-treatment, use the ball of the thumb. Press firmly on the roof of the mouth, as nearly as possible directly under the area where the pain is located. For example, if the pain is in the forehead, pressure should be made immediately over the roots of the front teeth. The pressure should be firm and steady and applied for five minutes. You might also apply pressure with the thumb and index finger in the indentation where the nose meets the eye sockets. Repeat as needed.

For cough or hoarseness, use the broad handle of a tablespoon as a tongue depressor. Pressure is usually applied at the center of the tongue, but if the irritation is extensive, pressure should also be applied to the extreme right and left side of the tongue. If the irritation seems to be low down in the bronchial tubes, apply pressure farther back on the tongue. Do this for three or four minutes at a time, and repeat every half-hour until relief is achieved. After six treatments, if there is no relief, stop.

For hoarseness or huskiness, combine the above action with the following, or use as an alternative. Grasp tongue firmly in a handkerchief and pull it forward as far as is comfortable. Slowly wriggle it from side to side for a few minutes.

For hiccups, grasp the tongue in a clean handkerchief and pull it forward, squeezing firmly at the same time. Hold while counting to one hundred.

For smarting, burning eyes or granulated lids, apply pressure to the upper joint and then the lower joint of the first and second fingers of the hand which corresponds to the eye involved. Then squeeze at the side of the finger so that the zone is sure to be completely covered. Broad rubber bands or tightly bound tapes may be used instead. If after five such treatments there is no relief, discontinue.

For itching and congestion of the eyelids, apply a bandage soaked with camphor water; wind it around the index finger.

For toothaches, but only until you can get to a dentist, grasp aching tooth firmly with the thumb and index finger immediately over the roots. Increase pressure until it becomes uncomfortable, release a slight bit, and hold firmly for four or five minutes.

For more information about zone therapy, write to Eunice D. Ingham, P.O. Box 948, Rochester, New York.

Dō-in is a relatively new variation of acupuncture, with a bit of zone therapy thrown in. It is a method of self-treatment and self-diagnosis intended to keep one in good health. It consists generally of rubbing and friction, light pounding, and gentle massage movements. There is a complete regimen, which includes a strict macrobiotic diet, intended to be followed each morning on rising, consisting mainly of brown rice, salt, sesame seeds, a few vegetables, and a little tea. The person practicing Dō-in is urged to follow a systematic diagnostic procedure each morning. For example, to test articulation, one hooks the fingers diagonally across the back. A slight to vigorous back-and-forth motion of the arms in this position is thought to stimulate the bladder, heart, small intestine, and lungs. Pressure applied on the inside of the right arm about five inches from the waist and about one-half inch in from the outer edge of the arm is supposed to stimulate or calm all other pressure points. One usually uses slow, deep pressure to calm, and light, rapid strokes to tonify. For more information, write to Happiness Press, 7557 Sunset Boulevard, Hollywood, California 90046.

Dr. Randolf Stone has spent some fifty years evolving polarity therapy, a mystical and highly complicated treatment. It is based on Oriental thought, principally accumulated during Dr. Stone's stay in India, where he was director of a clinic. His theory bears a striking resemblance to both yoga and acupuncture, but he uses manipulation and massage of a deep variety, much like that used in rolfing (see next chapter). Dr. Stone attempts to distribute "vital energy" (prana) and adjust so-called "polarity fields" so that the subject is in a proper position relative to gravity. One must know the ". . . anatomical relationships and functions as plus (+) and minus (−) energy polarities and be able to balance them by scientific skill." The plus-and-minus concept bears a resemblance to the Chinese yin and yang. This therapy involves a great deal of skill and study, and most or all practitioners are located on the West Coast. For those who are interested, I suggest writing for information to Pierre Pannetier, 401 North Glassell, Orange, California 92666.

8

The Body-Mind People

God guard me from the thoughts men think
In the mind alone.
He that sings a lasting song
Thinks in a marrow bone.
—*William Butler Yeats**

There are those in the healing arts "marching to a different drummer" from many of our parents or grandparents. This new breed of healers rejects the rigidly deterministic Cartesian logic of the philosopher René Descartes, who said, "I think, therefore I am."

Descartes reasoned, "I may have no *body*: this might be an illusion. But thought is different." This is rejected by these "body-mind people." They repudiate the alienation between body and mind and believe instead that the body and mind (or flesh and spirit) are inseparable, one, a "whole." Thus they reject putting the responsibility for the "body" strictly within the province of the physician, and the "mind" in the province of the psychiatrist.

This new movement came out of the existentialist philosophy of such men as Jean-Paul Sartre, who preferred, like Pascal, the "... heart's reasons which the reason knows not of." It also borrowed greatly from the theories of psychologist Wilhelm Reich (on muscular armor) and from the work on "body types" of

*"The King of the Great Clock Tower"

W.H. Sheldon. And it has to thank the ancient Oriental body arts such as hatha yoga, Tai Chi, and Zen awareness. For this book I concentrate mainly on the work of Ida Rolf, because it comes closest to what one usually thinks of as massage. Rolfers, as they are called, apply manual pressure and touch, usually while the subject is prone. Although chiropractors also do deep manipulation, sometimes in a way that looks like the Rolf technique, they work principally on manipulation of the spine, and they make no claims of resultant release of muscular armor and increased psychological freedom as rolfers do.

(Jefferson L. Sulzer, Ph.D., however, has written that "In contrast to some psychosomatic theories which stress the 'power of mind over body,' chiropractic tends to emphasize the importance of body in determining mental and emotional states. . . ." Dr. Sulzer points to the growing body of literature showing a strong relationship between tension of the body and anxiety, and, finally, disease; but this does not differ, except in emphasis, from the accepted medical viewpoint.)

What is Rolfing?

Now in her late seventies, Ida Rolf, the founder of "structural integration," or rolfing, is a Ph.D. biochemist and physiologist. For twelve years she was an associate in organic chemistry at the Rockefeller Institute, and for the past forty years she has been perfecting her techniques in the practice and teaching of her method. Most of the practitioners of rolfing have been trained and have settled in California at Esalen Institute in Big Sur. As of late 1972 there were only about fifty-five rolfers throughout the country, but their numbers are increasing so rapidly that the count is now much higher, and it is still growing. There is a large group of rolfers in Boulder, Colorado, and there are now some in the New York area.

How does it work? Whereas osteopaths manipulate the fascial tissue (connective tissue) in specific injured areas to relieve a particular injury, rolfing systematically manipulates the fascia of all the major muscles, using fists, fingers, elbows, or knees. It is done systematically with an extensive knowledge of the anatomy on the part of the rolfer. Anyone who becomes a rolfer must answer to a Guild of Structural Integrationists and meet certain requirements. About ten months of study are necessary in addition to the equivalent of two years of pre-med training and a license which states that the applicant has experience in "touching" people (chiropractor, physical therapist, masseur, etc.). A rolfer must be over twenty-five years old.

The entire rolfing procedure should take ten sessions. In the first session the chest and abdomen are manipulated. In subsequent sessions, the various muscle groups are stretched and the minute fibers (fibrils) that have formed between muscles are loosened; bunched tendons are freed, and shortened joints are made more elastic so they can move more freely. The person who has undergone rolfing should thus be able to move within the laws of gravity with greater economy and with a new grace.

During the manipulations, which are often painful, there is a deep emotional response, and old emotional traumas or physical pains are brought to the surface. This emotional response can occur during the session itself, when the subject may be moved to scream, cry, moan, or laugh. Or it may occur later, for seemingly no reason. Or it can appear in a dream. Rolfers claim that these are old pains which have been stored in the muscles and are freed when the muscular armor is released.

What do the structural integrationists hope to achieve? By reorganizing a person's fascial structure and realigning the entire body, the structural integrationists think that it is possible to reverse the effects of bodily disintegration. In so doing, they claim that they can restore resilience, grace, and economy of movement and relieve destructive muscular patterns.

Valerie Hunt of the University of California, Los Angeles, did a study on fourteen persons undergoing rolfing. She found, using electrical measurement of the muscles, that the activity of the nervous system involved in simple movements took shorter periods of active muscle contraction after a person was rolfed. This suggests that after rolfing there is less neuromuscular tension and more efficient use of energy. Another investigator, Julian Silverman, with the California Department of Mental Hygiene, worked with the same subjects, using electroencephalographs and computers to measure brain-wave patterns. He also did personality and biochemical tests. According to him, "the data from all our tests, combined with those from Dr. Hunt's study, seem to indicate that rolfing creates a more spontaneous, open, rhythmic reaction to the environment and to one's own kinesthetic and proprioceptive sensations."

Ida Rolf on Rolfing

Rolf began her independent work after twelve years as associate in organic chemistry at the Rockefeller Institute. It grew out of this scientific orientation at a time when, Dr. Rolf recalls, most everyone was convinced the living body was a law unto itself both physically and chemically. The body and mind were considered separate and unchanging dualities. Then once urea was synthesized in a test tube, our attitudes began to change. When more and more of the body's chemicals were synthesized, we started to accept that the body and mind are somewhat interrelated.

The first assumption that rolfers make is that "No matter what else a human being may be, he is certainly an aggregate of particles operating in a three-dimensional space and within the atmosphere of the earth. Therefore he is subject to the envelope of gravity which surrounds the earth, and as such he must obey certain physical laws of the universe." One such law is that bodies are plastic and "capable of being deformed continuously and permanently in any direction without rupture." This same plasticity which makes the living body vulnerable to deterioration, Dr. Rolf believes can be used to counteract deterioration and to rebuild a person's structure toward a more normal, anatomically efficient position with respect to gravity.

This may be achieved by making use of another law: Collagen (or connective tissue, called fascia when surrounding the muscles) has a very complicated protein chemistry, and " . . . it is such that we are able to change it." Ida Rolf explains that practitioners of structural integration believe that the substance responsible for the structure and support of the body is this collagen. "If you put pressure or energy onto that collagen, it changes its length, position, function and sometimes the disposition of the mineral element."

This is precisely the mechanism of rolfing. Rolfers work by applying pressure with their fists, fingers, elbows or knees to each one of the major muscles of the body. They often press deeply to loosen minute fibrils that have formed between muscles, to free bunched tendons and stretch shortened joints to make them more elastic and able to move more freely. They work as one might mould a sculpture. To Ida Rolf, the actual manipulative work with the fascia might be likened to an onion—layer lies within layer. Deeper layers are affected only as more superficial ones lose their rigidity. By manipulation of the fascia, the body is restructured toward a more anatomically efficient position. This produces more appropriate movement within gravity. The change in the structure is then made permanant through these new patterns of movement.

The ideal structure in a standing person is evaluated in terms of horizontal and vertical lines: an imaginary line is drawn through the ear, shoulder, hip bone, knee and ankle, and other horizontal lines arranged so the major weight blocks—the head, thorax, pelvis and legs—are distributed in a balanced manner.

An Interview with a Rolfer

Ida Rolf seems a formidible woman, and the demands on her time and energy are such that even a younger person would find them difficult to fulfill, so I decided to interview someone more easily accessible to fill in the gaps in my knowledge of rolfing. At a conference in which Dr. Rolf spoke, she credited a young rolfer, Owen James, with helping in her program. I asked him for an interview, to which he agreed.

The interview took place in his rambling New York upper west side apartment, casually decorated in "early Salvation Army" mixed with Oriental trappings and remnants of west coast living: some scenes of the rock-bound west coast were on the walls, wind chimes hung from the doors, and Japanese-style screens covered the windows. The outer door was kept ajar, with a sign posted for a visitor to knock before entering, and wind chimes signaled the door's opening—a small thing, but this indicated to me that the occupant was not a confirmed New York dweller; every New

Yorker I know has buzzers and locks on the doors and windows. In the living/waiting room there was a piano, music stand, reading material, and comfortable chairs; the atmosphere was relaxing. There was a note on the door suggesting that anyone who enters should remove his shoes, Oriental style.

As I waited for Owen to finish with someone he was seeing, I heard a few "ouches" emanating from the room in which he was working. He soon entered.

Owen James was slim, fair-skinned with rather long hair and a full moustache; I'd call him aesthetic-looking. He moved very silently and gracefully. There wasn't a trace of nervousness in his gestures or slouching. Ida Rolf's claim that her technique achieves "economy of movement" was well exemplified in the person of Owen James. I asked if he'd ever been a dancer. He answered that he hadn't, but that he did study it for a short while because his sister is a dancer, but that he was " . . . a professional flutist—a musician and a teacher, who always taught people to produce tones from their body." When I questioned his credentials as a rolfer, he said he had been a licensed masseur, he was trained in Gestalt therapy, and he had studied with Ida Rolf and had been "very rolfed" by her.

I asked Owen what kinds of people came to him for rolfing. He answered that there were people of all ages; he once worked with Ida on a five-month-old child, and he's worked on people in their seventies. They come to him for "every reason under the sun," he said, and when asked what kind of symptoms they had, he answered that he was not directly concerned with symptoms (much as in the Oriental philosophies) and that symptoms often go away spontaneously as the rolfer balances the body. During the course of our interview he said that people with chronic disorders such as hypertension and asthma could be helped by rolfing. I asked if he would treat someone with a fracture, and he answered, "not until the fracture healed." If it did not heal after some time had elapsed, that would be a different case, for he did once treat someone with a fracture that had not healed after a period of years.

I suppose all of us who hear about rolfing for the first time are most intrigued with the notion that pain is "inflicted." I was particularly curious, because somewhere in the back of my mind I was toying with the idea of trying one or two sessions myself. Owen did agree that rolfing hurts. But he claimed that the pain was not inflicted by the rolfer putting pressure on a certain place, but rather the pain " ... is already in your body from early childhood." He sees rolfing as an "unraveling." "It's as if you were a novel and your entire history were there in your body." (Owen doesn't consider the body and mind as separate.) "As I go through the tissues with my hands—in the fascia—it's the same thing to me as if I opened the pages of a book. . . . If the subject is able, or willing, to focus into his body, he becomes 'one' with the body and is able to see his life history there. . . . This is a difficult thing for most people. It sometimes happens spontaneously at the moment of rolfing, and sometimes it happens hours afterward. Sometimes it takes days for certain traumas to come to consciousness. Sometimes it happens the instant I put my hand on a person. If one is focused into the part of the body where I am working, the person may experience a little pain, on the one hand. On the other hand, he will experience complete relief."

I asked what he meant by "release," and what he described sounded very Reichian to me. He said that the pain one experiences during rolfing is already there in the body and that rolfers believe they are affecting "body armor"; thus they are affecting repressed memories. They believe that their process "raises energy from the person which he needs to be able to become a more 'whole' person." He continued that rolfing "is a very systematic, a very organized, and a highly skilled art." (He stressed the word "art.") And he said that they deal "at a specific level . . . at a specific time . . . for a specific person." What I believe he meant by that was that every person has his own tempo, and rolfers work slightly differently with every individual, of course within a certain basic rule structure. I find this stressing of individual "uniqueness" a very positive statement, because I have a personal bias against the therapies (both physical and psychological) in which the so-called therapist attempts to "impose" a theoretical concept upon a person rather than let the subject go at his own pace and in his own style.

What did he and the rolfers mean when they spoke of "energy"? "Energy is a misused word," he stressed, "for it is used to classify many different things, including 'blocked' energy and 'freed' energy. . . . The acupuncturist speaks of 'life energy,' the spirit healer or psychic speaks of another kind of energy. It may be that they are all referring to the same kind of energy, which they deal with in different ways and at different levels. Some people may also have different sensitivities to it."

The conversation was taking a mystical turn, much to my liking, and so I asked a favorite question: did he see an "aura" around people? He said he sometimes did, and that the auras were sometimes in color. Since he seemed not to want to pursue the subject, I dropped it. (In the introduction I mention that by Kirlian photography one can see what some claim to be an "aura," or that emanation of energy which is thought to surround all living objects and which can be made to change color and shape.)

As I was thinking that I might try rolfing myself, I asked some questions to allay my fears. I asked if it could be dangerous for a person who didn't know what he was doing to work on the body. Owen said he thought it might be, because there are certain rules that "have been handed down for thousands of years," and every practitioner should follow these. I asked if he meant to include the rule that one should always massage in the direction of the veins or heart. He agreed that was one, and then he mentioned another: Acupuncturists claim that the "life energy" moves up the spine, and so when massaging on the spinal cord, one should move upward. Otherwise, one should move downward when massaging on the back. Most of these laws "work the same way that acupuncture laws work."

Since he was relating rolfing to other forms of therapy, I thought I'd try to put rolfing in context with other healing arts. I asked Owen what he thought about some other forms of treatment. He said that if he himself were sick he would see a chiropractor if there wasn't a rolfer around. As far as osteopathy is concerned, he mentioned that many of them work more on surface muscles, and "they don't always take into account the whole body. For example, if a person has a bad knee, they might just work on the knee. But if the bad knee is the result of a twisted pelvis, no matter how many times the knee is fixed locally, the trouble will still remain."

I wondered then about the permanence of rolfing. Once a person was rolfed, wouldn't he slip back? Owen claimed that it wasn't usually the case. "But if a person falls down the stairs, it might throw the body out of alignment. Or if a person has an automobile accident, for example." I wondered more about this ideal state in relation to gravity. Did Owen think there was any person who didn't require rolfing? He didn't think so, he said, "for we are not born standing. . . . When we learn to walk, we do so to some extent by watching others walk—our mother, our brother, and so forth. . . .

A baby walks the way it *can* walk." Then he talked about how a child might also have accidents—fall out of the crib, fall out of trees—and all these things might throw him out of balance. He also mentioned that walking on high heels might throw a girl off balance.

I was still puzzled about this ideal state and about what I had once heard Ida Rolf say at a meeting—that rolfers were making "superior beings." Some psychotherapists at the meeting clearly took offense to that, probably because some of them were old enough to remember the Second World War and the concept of "Aryan superiority." Owen said he wanted to make it really clear what Ida Rolf meant by that, because he was aware that many people misunderstood. "She feels that rolfing is a technique by itself that releases emotions and that changes the physical body into a higher state of consciousness, into a 'new man.' She feels she is making a new person, that is, a person with a new level of functioning. . . . Her meaning of superior people, then, is making a man (or woman) that is more toward the apex."

"What about when she talks of making 'patterned' bodies?" I asked.

"There are certain laws in the system of man and the universe which prove that if you take any kind of system which is built around a balanced organized space, you will get a system that is using less energy and which is able therefore to work at a higher level." He stressed this, then paused. "You have more blood flowing. You take in more oxygen. You use less energy. So that means you can do more things and are into a higher state of 'being.' In other words, instead of always *having* to do things, always *having* to hold yourself up, you are in a balanced state like building blocks which are built on top of each other and are all symmetrical. Gravity, then, which works at right angles to the earth, will not act as a destructive force but will act as a tool which runs right through that line of balance, or symmetry. . . . Then you will not have to work at forcing yourself up, but you will simply retain a state of support in which your 'being' can then bloom. . . . All of that, I believe, is what Ida Rolf means when she speaks of making a 'new man.' She is restructuring people to automatically stand erect within gravity."

Essentially the entire meaning of rolfing is this: "What we are doing is *creating a new man in different motion*, and when we create a new motion, we create a new man."

He paused for effect. Then he spoke about how eighty percent of our motion is *contractive* motion. "Fear, anxiety, strain, shock—all of these are contractive. Walking down a street in New York requires contractive motion. . . . Take the young people today—the sixteen-to-twenty-year-olds—you see them with shoulders in, head forward, like this." (He pulled his head down, chest in and shoulders up.) "This is certainly not the result of a society which is experiencing openness, freedom of expression, expansion of oneself. It's the opposite. . . . I believe Ida is saying that she can make a new man and thereby make a new society. . . . By changing the movements that are made in a society, you can actually start to change the society. If eighty percent of our motion is contractive, then you will produce a contractive society. If you change the motions by changing the habit patterns of the body as rolfers do, you can start to change the way a society thinks and functions."

I felt this was a dramatic point to stop at. I concluded with arranging a session for myself. I wanted about five sessions to get a good idea of how it felt to be rolfed. Owen wasn't quite willing to go along with only a few sessions, since rolfing's object is total balance within gravity. I managed to persuade him that since a few sessions couldn't hurt, we'd start out with plans for five sessions and then see what happened.

I had a few fears. I asked Owen if there could be any danger of a heart attack due to the pain if an older person is predisposed to it. "The opposite is true," he said, and he mentioned that Fritz Perls was rolfed by Ida when he was close to seventy and felt that it had added years to his life. He also told of his father, who had a heart attack and was kept alive when Ida did some rolfing on him. I later checked with an osteopath and with Dr. Liberson of the V.A. hospital in Miami, Florida, as to whether there could be any physical harm from this form of treatment. Dr. Liberson stated that as far as he knows there have been "no accidents connected with this form of deep connective tissue massage," but he feels "it should be practiced with great knowledge of the tissues involved." Because rolfers receive sufficient training in anatomy and manual techniques, I felt reassured. I looked forward to my rolfing experience nervously but with enthusiasm.

I've Been Rolfed and I Feel Fine

In preparing this book, I embarked on a new "body trip" when I agreed to be rolfed. But it has all been worth it now that I've completed ten rolfing sessions, for I feel better than ever before. My body moves in new and better ways, and I have a greater "awareness." For you to understand what these changes are and what they mean to me, I must tell you a few personal things about myself. You won't hear of anything so dramatic as arthritis "miraculously healed" (which I'm told does happen during rolfing), because I'm in relatively good health except for some assorted aches and pains and certain bodily limitations which my periodic yoga sessions have caused me to notice. The discoveries

I've made have been somewhat intangible, often theoretical, and mostly quite subjective.

A few more personal facts: I'm a New Yorker, and consequently riddled with ever-present tensions, in the subways, at work, in the street. I'm in a competitive type of work as a writer and photographer—hence more tension; and my work requires that I sit too much of the time. At forty, I'm single and I come from a Jewish middle-class environment, with whatever defects or advantages are inherent in this. I have a tendency to overeat, and I'm about ten pounds overweight. Lately it seems I rarely "date," and the resources available to single people I usually find objectionable. I don't enjoy excessive drinking in "singles" bars, and I shyly admit I often "tense up" when meeting new people. About twelve years ago I ended a three-year course of psychoanalysis and group therapy.

This is the person who embarked upon rolfing. So far, these externals haven't changed, although I am experiencing a new awareness of my feelings, which are being modified somewhat in relation to these "facts" of my life. For one thing, I feel softer, less "edgy," and less defensive. When I do become defensive, I can express it more openly, and I am more aware of it and how to cope with it. I walk and sit straighter, and I look better. My new "straighter" self feels better to me, and I even feel I'm beginning to want to establish new, more intimate relationships. Here is a "play-by-play" account of my rolfing—my thoughts and feelings.

November 8, 1972, 10:00 A.M. My first rolfing session. It was very powerful. The instant my chest was touched, however lightly, I felt a strong fear of death. This was a new feeling to me and one which I had not been in touch with before. And I believe this fear of death was a "real" fear—that I was fearing the loss of all the old habits and patterns which would cause the old "me" to die. The emotion made me scream and cry out, and it seemed I made a terribly loud sound, although Owen claimed it was nothing at all, barely audible. I continued to experience this fear of death each time a particular place on my chest was touched.

I lay on a bed parallel to a floor-to-ceiling mirror, where I could glimpse myself from time to time. It was a shock looking at my unclothed body, as it was a shock at first taking my clothes off. (Sometime during the course of these sessions I was to begin to like my body and the way it looked—a seemingly small thing, but to me a great accomplishment.)

At the end of the first session, Owen showed me in the mirror how I was now able to take deeper breaths than ever before. It looked to me as if my entire upper chest had miraculously opened up, and my breathing was indeed deeper and fuller.

In retrospect, on November 14. During the week I felt an even more intense craving to eat the wrong foods. There was a lingering pain in my chest until yesterday. It is strange, but my yoga session was worse; it was harder to sit up and touch my toes. One thing was good, though; I seemed to have more breath than usual. The first interesting emotional change occurred today. I received an upsetting telephone call. Instead of just pacing up and down as I usually do, although I did pace, when I felt the tension in my throat and chest, I moved my arms up and out and flailed about with them and emitted a scream. This helped; after a few minutes the anxiety subsided completely and I felt fresh and free again. I conclude that because of the rolfing I was now able to release this emotion rather than suppress it within my body in tightening and tensing as I would have before. This, I believe, is a healthier pattern, and it's new to me.

November 16, 1972. Rolfing session number two. Owen worked mostly on my legs and feet. There was little pain here. In the early part of the session I consciously held my emotions back and cut myself off from my feelings, because I was aware there were other people in the house and I was embarrassed and didn't want to make too much noise. In other words, I was trying to be a "good girl," as I always did as a child, a response which in this case as an adult no longer served me well. Here was a useful emotional insight! Owen said my feet were like rubber, and not well grounded, and he just couldn't get hold of my muscles. He recommended that when I take a bath at night I massage my feet and rub oil on them. (I've been doing this, and it has improved my feet.) Owen also pointed out that, in fact, I have "weak knees," and this is also an emotional attitude. Afterward I felt somewhat more in contact with the ground as I walked, and I also felt that my weight was more evenly distributed. He also worked on my tense back muscles and my shoulders. It felt good and made me laugh, which was a nice feeling, as I don't laugh often enough.

I asked Owen, "If, as rolfers claim, the pain one feels during rolfing is only one's 'own pain' and not pain which the rolfer imposes on you, then it must follow that you [Owen], who have been 'very rolfed,' will no longer feel pain when someone presses deeply into your connective tissue during rolfing." Owen said that was true. He said for the longest time he had terrible pain under his armpits, inside his mouth, and in his chest during each rolfing session. Then one day Ida said, "That's enough of that," and she worked on these areas for some time. The pain has since stopped, he says. Personally, I'm not quite convinced of the "your-own-pain" theory. But I can't reject rolfing as a result of my doubts, because so far I have felt emotionally freer after each session, and more "alive."

During the week of November 17–23rd. Yesterday I met Elaine L., whom I haven't seen for over a year.

When I first stopped her, she didn't recognize me at all. During our conversation she kept trying to put her finger on what was different about me. Was it my hair? "Yes," she said, "I think it was redder. . . . Maybe that's it. Or maybe you've lost weight." And so on. Both of these are true. But could it be it's my attitude that is different, and that this is due to the rolfing?

Another thing happened during this week that precipitated a revelation of sorts. I was held up at knifepoint. Afterward I thought about my reactions. I never looked at the man in the face or eyes. I unconsciously slumped physically, as if trying to bore a hole through the floor so I could slip right through and disappear. Later I could hardly give a description of the man, even though he was right in front of me for a good four minutes. I realize this may be a common enough reaction if a person is frightened, but it is also self-defeating, as a person in such a physical attitude cannot defend himself. One should ideally be more like the cat at rest, who even while completely relaxed can respond with quick and decisive movements. When frightened, a cat puts its back up and readies itself for defensive action. Also, by not looking at the aggressor, one cannot really know who the enemy is, nor receive or send out eye signals. I vowed to somehow build greater confidence in my strength and to keep my body "toned" and in readiness, as a cat.

November 24, 1972. Session number three. During the session there was some pain. Owen worked on my back, hips, and side. One area around my torso felt so exquisitely painful I asked if an "organ" weren't there. He laughed and showed me how lightly he was touching, and when he had me open my eyes and look at where he was working, I realized, of course, there were no organs in the area, for he was pressing lightly under my ribs around my waist. I must have been feeling my own tension, and perhaps some stored emotional pain. This is a very vulnerable area for me, and I must undo my old habit of "slumping" when I sit or work. Once I thought this was relaxing, but now I realize it is not. After the session, I generally felt more stretched through the waistline and torso, where well I need it.

Owen talked about how really noisy the body can be—about the "squoonches" and "squeaks"—and I remembered how he would start to laugh as my leg bones would crack. He said he often thought how wonderful it would be to sit where there are no other sounds and concentrate only on the sound of the blood moving through the body. He claims he is able to "think" his weight up or down about four pounds. I suppose this is theoretically possible, since Indian fakirs can lie on a bed of nails, and the miracle of self-hypnosis does exist. Also, the new alpha training shows that the mind can indeed change the physiological workings of the body.

During our sessions Owen also concentrates a great deal on my breathing, and he has told me that ultimately I will be able, like him, to feel my breath moving from the top of my head to the tip of my toes. He has pointed to the small of my back or at a spot above and between my buttocks and says that I will be able to feel my breath to there.

November 30, 1972. Rolfing session number four. During the week I was feeling a new awareness of my "powers" and a kindness toward them, and I had the feeling that I really "owned" myself. This is a complicated sensation which I won't go into detail about here; but let me tell you, the feeling of "owning" oneself is a very good sensation, and power, contrary to what one might think, is a softening influence. I was softer. Perhaps Rollo May is right when he says that it is not power, but powerlessness which corrupts. But today, for some reason, I felt weak, tired. I slept soundly for eleven hours last night. Perhaps this is because of the radical changes working in my body. Owen worked on my legs again. This time I discovered a very painful area on the top of the leg. After the session I felt a tingling and a new contact with parts of my legs that had been deadened. I felt in greater contact with the ground. My earlier "blue" feeling disappeared.

December 1–4. I have given in to being sick and depressed for the past few days. I slumped around and stayed in bed. Maybe I'm coming down with a "bug," or maybe some emotional wounds are opening up. I have no idea. I know in retrospect that I did "give in" to a feeling that I might have fought with my new bodily awareness, and "giving in" to these depressions and feeling guilty about this lethargy is a part of my old pattern.

December 5, 1972. Rolfing session number five. This session made me feel better. Owen worked on my abdomen and the front of my torso. My body turned red and stayed that way for a few hours. My arms were tingling, and so was my lower abdomen, where he worked. This was a new sensation in an area where I rarely have any feeling. While I lay down he gave me a good sensory exercise, which has since helped my breathing. He told me to imagine I am breathing in cold, bubbling spring water to the back of the lungs. I had another revelation: I overeat to choke down feelings, and I get energy, while I really need instead to get more energy from "within."

December 6, 1972. I went to my usual yoga session, and I noticed that my body is different now, and it is better. I am now able to do "the fish"—backward-bending pose—and I feel that more vertebrae of my spine are beginning to "give" so I can bend backward. On the other hand, I'm worse at another pose—the one in which I bend forward and touch my toes while in a sitting position. I must ask Owen why!

December 10, 1972. My neighbor Sally S. remarked on how well I look. I've also been noticing that now I can move my pelvis forward to do the rock-'n'-roll motions that I never could do comfortably before. Before rolfing I could do only the side-to-side hip motions of the rumba, which always made me feel "dated." I danced in front of the mirror and was delighted at my "freer" pelvis. Clothes fit me differently. I can now tuck blouses in my slacks or skirts, whereas because of my thick waistline I always used to wear overblouses—anything to "hide" my body, particularly my torso. Now, while I'm still not "Miss America" material, my body is mine and I accept it. And it does look somewhat better since it has been stretched through the middle.

December 13 and 14. I woke up on December 13 with terrible muscle cramps in my left shoulder, neck, and arm, which lasted most of the day. I've also been overeating for a few days. On December 14 I felt depressed and started to slump into a "decline." At one point during the day I felt my left leg vibrating.

December 15, 1972. Rolfing session number six. Owen worked on my back. It was a marvelous session. I cooperated well by putting my consciousness where he worked. I felt very much in touch with my legs afterward. Owen claims the reason I couldn't do the toe touching from a sitting position in yoga was because my back muscles still need work and my hamstring muscles are tense. He had me sit in a position to do the exercise as he worked on the muscles that were holding me back. Owen claims the pain I had on the thirteenth was because of old emotional reactions in dreams which my "new" rolfed body could no longer accept. He said the same thing happened to him during his rolfing.

January 10, 1973. Rolfing session number seven. As it has been some time since my last session, I was a little apprehensive. I had almost forgotten how good these sessions usually make me feel in the long run. This time Owen worked on my back, neck, and face. The work on my face was pleasant and relaxing. He also worked on the muscles of my back again, so I was able to get into the yoga position, and for the first time I could bend over my legs so that my torso was pressed flat against my legs and my hands clasped my ankles. Owen worked a lot on my neck and shoulders to get my shoulders down, for I hold them too high. I was able to breathe deeper, and he gave me another useful exercise. He told me to breathe as deeply as I thought I could; then, when my lungs were as full as I thought I could get them, he told me to take in some more breath, then still some more. It worked. He said that part of the reason I didn't breathe deeply was because I thought I couldn't. He told me to breathe deeply, starting from the back of the ribs, while I kept my ribs and back still flat on the table. "Our back gives us strength," he said. All of this was helpful, and I made the observation that before my sessions I had little consciousness of my back, and most of my awareness was focused on my front. Owen also showed me a better position to hold my arms. He told me to "think myself wide." I laughed, because I felt that I wanted to be thin rather than wide. But he said that thinking myself wide will not make me fatter, only help me to feel my strength and hold my body better and more centered with gravity. Also, since my torso is so heavy-muscled, he asked me to try to "think" these muscles stringier and finer. He said it would take some time, but it could work. I noticed another thing; generally, rolfing makes me feel more planted in earth. After I got home I had to take a nap, and I did little for the rest of the day. I wonder what is now at work within. . . .

January 16, 1973. Rolfing session number eight. This was the most powerful and painful session of all. Owen worked inside my mouth. With each spot he pressed there was a different sensation; pressure on one particular place on the lower inside of my mouth caused much deep-throated screaming; in another spot, the cries of a child. I recalled how as a child my mother used to always tell me to "close my mouth," and my anger at her was still there. I also recalled her favorite taunt: "Children should be seen and not heard." Owen said the mouth is a painful area for many people; it was for him. This is because many people hold back emotions in their mouth and jaw. He also pressed my tongue down and showed me that I hold the back of my tongue up and how it would be better if I held it down. He agreed that perhaps this may be related to why I tend to overeat. Finally, when I felt a very painful area in my mouth start to "give way" after his prodding and pressing, I found myself saying, "I feel like a grown-up." I was jolted by this utterance. It was true. I felt reborn. While my mouth was being rolfed, I also noticed an abrupt and immediate improvement in my vision; everything became clearer. Owen said that had happened to him as well. When the session ended, I felt like a more loving and sensual adult.

January 17, 1973. Today I went to the dentist. It was a miracle how relaxed I was in spite of the fact that I had to have a crown put on my tooth. I almost fell asleep in the chair, and I had to ask the dentist if he hadn't put a tranquilizer in the Novocain; he hadn't. I can think of no answer other than that the rolfing had freed me of my usual nervousness.

January 19, 1973. Rolfing session number nine. Owen worked on my legs. The evening before, I had had dinner with my parents, and today my legs were weak. It seems when I sit back and don't take a stand, as had occurred the evening before, I do something physically with my legs.

February 2, 1973. My tenth session. Owen worked on my legs again, on my sides and torso, and my arms and back. He found that painful area around my waistline again. How do I feel now that rolfing has been "completed"? I feel I will probably need to go back again occasionally for a few sessions from time to time. I will continue doing yoga, for I feel strongly that everyone needs some body work, and particularly someone who is as sedentary as I am. I believe this remains true throughout one's lifetime, as everyone's body is always changing.

I now feel I am more able to "take a stand." But still, like anyone, I occasionally feel sad, have pains, and am depressed; but I believe I know better how to handle it. For if a person knows *why* she is depressed, it lessens the impact of the depression. Further, I generally am more "open," and I feel more like a full-grown sensual adult woman.

The Alexander Technique

> It is impossible fully to describe the benefits both in health and *joie de vivre* which I owed, and still owe, to this radical alteration in my physique; for although nothing could of course correct my consti-

tutional failings, I was a changed man. . . . It has certainly prolonged my life.*

What, exactly, is the Alexander technique? Getting up, sitting down, walking, standing, shutting windows, reaching for a pencil, tying a shoelace—*all* of our usual activities, from the most strenuous to the simplest, involve us in complicated patterns of movement and rest that, for better or for worse, constitute our particular use of ourselves. According to Alexander, we must acquire a better use of ourselves, particularly those of us who suffer back pain, excessive fatigue, poor posture, or physical tension. This better pattern of habits necessitates the greatest lengthening of the spine possible in whatever we do. Alexander called this vertebral lengthening in activity "the true and primary movement" in each and every act. He later called it "primary control." This is the classic threefold pattern that is the basis of all Alexander work (and it is not as simple as it seems: "(1) Let the neck be free (which means merely to see that you do not increase the muscle tension of the neck in any act); (2) Let the head go forward and up—forward for the neck, that is, not forward in space (which means that you see that you do not tense the neck muscles by pulling the head back or down in any act); (3) Let the torso lengthen and widen out (which means that you see that you do not shorten and narrow the back by arching the spine)."

These directions are achieved at first with the help of an Alexander teacher, who sometimes uses a light touch to guide the student as he develops a "kinesthetic sense" of a better way of moving and "being."

Alexander technique requires "concentrated thought," and the student first must "... make a conscious

* A. M. Ludovisi, describing his course of Alexander work, quoted in *The Resurrection of the Body: The Writings of F. Matthias Alexander* (selected and introduced by Edward Maisel), New York, Delta, 1969.

decision to *do nothing*. The teacher then presents him with a series of verbal directions . . ." (such as "Let the neck be free") ". . . which the student repeats to himself." In the process the teacher often uses her hands to give the student a kinesthetic experience of his own body and to show him how he uses it and how he might use it better. The amount and kind of touch that is applied varies according to the teacher, but usually it is a very light finger pressure.

Who was F. M. Alexander? F. Matthias Alexander was an Australian actor who began his body work when, in the 1880's, while on stage, he suddenly lost his voice. His doctor told him not to speak for a while and his voice would return. Alexander followed instructions; his voice did return. He began to work again, but he soon lost his voice again. He rested, and it returned. This continued; he would lose his voice, doctors would tell him to rest it (for that was all they knew how to do), and so on. This was no way for an actor to live, and so Alexander, being an enterprising man, took matters into his own hands. As George Bernard Shaw, who was later to become his student, wrote, he had the true scientific spirit and industry, and so he set himself to discovering what it was that he was really doing to disable himself in this fashion. Alexander started to study his body minutely in the mirror. He noticed that his body moved in certain ways as he spoke. For one thing, he would pull his head back and push his neck forward. During this prolonged observation period of about nine or ten years he reeducated his body to new patterns of movement, and thereby he regained his voice permanently and developed a complete technique. Alexander emerged with the conviction that mind and body are an inseparable whole.

Alexander's work impressed the well-known surgeon Dr. J. W. Steward McKay, who tried the technique on some patients and found that it could be used in certain gynecological conditions instead of surgery. The doctor encouraged Alexander to go to London and make his technique known, which he did. Thereafter it became the "darling" of many performing artists of the time, such as Sir Henry Irving and Constance Collier. Prominent physicians took it up, and influential figures in America: John Dewey, Lewis Mumford, Waldo Frank, and J. B. Duke, to mention a few.

Who uses Alexander technique? They are referred to as "students" by Alexander teachers, and they fall into three general categories: "(1) those who must use their bodies with maximum ease and effectiveness: actors, dancers, singers, athletes, musicians; (2) those whose carriage is bad, uncomfortable, or even painful, or whose occupation causes bad postural habits; (3) those with medical problems. Pupils frequently are referred to Alexander teachers by physicians, because physical disability that has been intensified through faulty body use results in an unnecessary increase in pain and fatigue."

At the Institute of Rehabilitative Medicine in New York, the technique has been used to help alleviate some cases of low backache, pinched nerve, scoliosis, tension syndrome, and certain other distortions. Dr. Allen Russek, director of specialized services there, explains that such means can be also used, on occasion, "as a substitute for such mechanical devices as halters, corset, neck braces, or shoulder pins: that is to say, in cases where it is possible to effect a change in the patient's center of gravity through internal shifting rather than external pressure."

To get more information, write to the American Center for the Alexander Technique, 142 West End Avenue, New York, New York 10024.

Imagined Massage: The Work of Dr. Moshe Feldenkrais

Dr. Feldenkrais's good record of rehabilitation in Israel has started to attract the attention of the world. He does not "treat," but he "teaches," and his highly evolved system has some similarity to Alexander theory. In his words, "There are two states of existence: waking and sleeping. Awareness is the third state, and in this state the individual knows exactly what he is doing while awake, just as we sometimes know when awake what we dreamed while asleep." For example, "at forty a man may become aware that one of his legs is shorter than the other, only after having suffered backaches, having had X rays. . . ." As we all know through personal experience, this is not only possible, but common. Feldenkrais claims it is possible "because the waking state in general more resembles sleep than awareness. . . ."

Four components make up the waking state: sensation, feeling, thought, and movement. By "sensation" he means to include the often neglected kinesthetic sense as well as the other five senses. Under the category of "feeling" he includes such emotions as "self-respect, inferiority, supersensitivity," as well as the usual emotions. "Thinking" includes all the functions of the intellect. "Movement" includes all temporal and spatial changes, such as "breathing, eating, speaking, blood circulation, and digestion." So Feldenkrais's definition of movement is broader than what one would normally imagine, and using movement is one way in which he increases a person's awareness. As he considers breathing a movement, he works a great deal on breathing. To show what his work is like, I include an example of some suggested exercises to increase a person's awareness of parts of the body of which he is customarily unconscious. It might be called "imagined massage."

Lie on your stomach and stretch your legs in such a way that they are symmetrical to the spine. Place one hand on top of the other on the ground in front of your head. Rest your forehead on the top hand. Now imagine that someone is pressing a finger on the heel of your right foot, which moves up the back of your calf to the knee. The pressure makes you feel the hardness of your leg bones. The imagined finger moves steadily and does not slip to the right or left.

Still lying on the stomach, try to imagine an iron ball rolling along your leg from the middle of the heel to the knee and back again. Try to identify in your mind all the points along the ball's path to make sure none are skipped. Continue imagining as the ball rolls from the knee to the thigh and to the buttock. Try to find where the ball would roll if you lifted your leg. Go on rolling the ball back to the knee and the heel and then back to the buttock.

Stretch your left arm forward. Keep it comfortably bent at the elbow. Then imagine the same heavy iron ball resting on the back of your hand. Find the spot where the ball could rest without falling, and then try to roll it toward the elbow. Imagine the exact, firm course along which it would roll to the elbow and back. Then imagine the same movement with someone's finger running along the arm. Continue in the same way from elbow to shoulder. Return the ball to the back of the hand; do the same for the imagined finger. Then imagine the ball first and then the finger moving from the back of the hand to the shoulder and the shoulderblade.

Conclusion

When I started this book I preferred not to stress any particular massage technique over another. As the work progressed, however, my knowledge and insights grew, so that I began to experience biases. As I feel it is impossible—even unwise—to hide one's point of view, I did not. I was careful, though, to give some discussion of every healing art that employs what might be called "massage." (It should include some kneading, pressing, or stroking, no matter how slight the touch or how seldom it's used.)

My overall conclusion is that massage is generally a useful technique for one to use on oneself or on a partner to enhance awareness, communication, sensual pleasure, and health. It helps to increase circulation, aid relaxation, and get more energy flowing—all of which means improved health and vitality.

Suggested Reading List

BODY-MIND TECHNIQUES

ALEXANDER, F. Matthias. *The Resurrection of the Body.* Selected and introduced by Edward Maisel. New York: Delta, 1971.

FELDENKRAIS, Moshe. *Awareness Through Movement.* New York and London: Harper & Row, 1972.

GENERAL MASSAGE

BEARD, G., and Wood, E. E. *Massage, Principles and Techniques.* Philadelphia and London: W. B. Saunders Company, 1964.

DOWNING, George. *The Massage Book.* California and New York: Random House, 1972.

ORIENTAL MEDICINE AND ORIENTAL METHODS OF MASSAGE

The Yellow Emperor's Classic of Internal Medicine; The Huang Ti Nei Ching Su Wen. Translated by Ilza Veith. Berkeley, Los Angeles, London: University of California Press, 1972.

MANN, Felix. *The Ancient Chinese Art of Healing.* New York: Random House, 1963.

PALOS, Stephen. *The Chinese Art of Healing.* New York: Herder & Herder; and Bantam Books, 1972.

PHILOSOPHY AND PSYCHOLOGY

HOWARD, Jane. *Please Touch.* New York: McGraw-Hill Book Co.; and Dell Publishing Co., 1971.

HUXLEY, Aldous. *The Art of Seeing.* New York and London: Harper & Brothers, 1942.

———. *The Perennial Philosophy.* New York and London: Harper & Brothers, 1945.

MAY, Rollo. *Power and Innocence*. Norton, 1972.
———, Ernest Angel, and Henry F. Ellenberger, eds. *Existence. A New Dimension in Psychiatry and Psychology*. New York: Basic Books, 1959.
PERLS, Frederick S., M.D., Ph.D. *Gestalt Therapy Verbatim*. Moab, Utah: Real People Press; and New York: Bantam Books, 1972.
REICH, Wilhelm. *Character Analysis*. 3rd ed. New York: The Noonday Press, 1961.
———. *The Function of the Orgone*, 2 vols. New York: Orgone Institute Press, 1948.
YUTANG, Lin. *The Wisdom of Lao Tse*. New York: Random House (Modern Library), 1948.

SELF-EXAMINATION

FRANKFORT, Ellen. *Vaginal Politics*. New York: Quadrangle Books, 1972.

UNORTHODOX MEDICINE

INGLIS, Brian. *The Case for Unorthodox Medicine*. New York: G. P. Putnam's Sons, 1965.

ZONE THERAPY

FITZGERALD, Wm. H., and Bowers, Edwin. *Zone Therapy*. Columbus, Ohio: I. W. Long, 1917. (Reprinted by Health Research, 70 Lafayette Street, Mokelumne Hill, California 95245).

OTHER BODY THERAPIES

ENELOW, Gertrude. *Body Dynamics*. New York: Citadel Press, 1963.
MENSENDIECK, Bess M. *Look Better, Feel Better*. New York and Evanston: Harper & Row, 1954.
TODD, Mabel Elsworth. *The Thinking Body. A Study of the Balancing Forces of Dynamic Man*. Paul B. Hoeber, Inc. 1937. (Republished by Dance Horizons, Incorporated, 1801 East 26th Street, Brooklyn, New York).

General Bibliography

American Medical Association: *Handbook of Massage and Physical Therapy*. Chicago: A.M.A.

"On Touching and Smelling." *Glamour*, January 1972, p. 82.

The Physiologic Basis of Osteopathic Medicine. Adapted from the symposium presented on October 7, 1967. New York: The Postgraduate Institute for Osteopathic Medicine and Surgery. 1970.

BARR, J. S., and Taslitz, N. "The Influence of Back Massage on Autonomic Functions," *Physical Therapy* 50: 1678–1691, 1970.

CASTANEDA, Carlos. *A Separate Reality*. New York: Simon and Schuster; and Pocket Books, 1972.

DINTENFASS, Julius. *Chiropractic. A Modern Way to Health*. New York: Pyramid Books, 1970.

DUNBAR, Flanders. *Mind and Body: Psychosomatic Medicine*. New York: Random House, 1955.

FRANK, H. *et al. Handbook of Physical Medicine and Rehabilitation*. Philadelphia and London: W. B. Saunders & Co., 1971.

HALL, Edward T. *The Hidden Dimension*. Doubleday & Company; and Garden City, New York: Anchor Books, 1969.

HARTLEY, Joel, M.D. *New Ways in First Aid*. Hart Publishing Co., Inc., 1971.

INKELES, G., and Todris, M. *The Art of Sensual Massage*. San Francisco: Straight Arrow Books, 1972.

KEEN, S. "Sing the Body Electric," *Psychology Today*, October 1970.

LAMB, Lawrence E., M.D. *Your Heart and How to Live with It*. New York: The Viking Press, 1969.

DE LANGRE, Jacques. *The First Book of Dō-in*. Hollywood, California: Happiness Press, 1971.

LOWEN, Alexander, M.D. *Physical Dynamics of Character Structure. Bodily Form and Movement in Analytic Therapy.* New York and London: Grune & Stratton, 1958.

MACKAY, Charles. *Extraordinary Popular Delusions and the Madness of Crowds.* Boston: L. C. Page & Company, 1932.

REMSEN, Guy. *Wake Up Your Body!* New York: David McKay Company, 1969.

RUSSELL, Bertrand. *A History of Western Philosophy.* New York: Simon & Schuster, 1945.

SERIZAWA, Katsusuke, M.D. *Massage. The Oriental Method.* Tokyo and San Francisco: Japan Publications, Inc., 1972.

SLAUGHTER, Frank S. *Your Body and Your Mind.* New York: New American Library, 1953.

STRAUS, Erwin. *The Primary World of Senses. A Vindication of Sensory Experience.* Straus, 1963.

TIDY, N. M. *Massage and Remedial Exercises in Medical and Surgical Conditions.* 3rd ed. Baltimore: William Wood & Co., 1937.

WATTS, Alan W. *The Way of Zen.* New York: New American Library, 1959.

ABOUT THE AUTHOR

After an early career as an actress, CONSTANCE YOUNG spent two years in the Speech and Drama Department of Syracuse University, then transferred to Columbia University, where she majored in science while working as a technician at Columbia University Presbyterian Hospital. She then worked as a medical writer for a Swiss pharmaceutical company in Westchester, New York. Since 1971 she has worked as a free-lance writer of scripts, books and articles on health and related subjects. Ms. Young has maintained a parallel career as a photographer whose work has been shown in several galleries (including the Architectural League and Soho Photo galleries in New York) and has been published in textbooks and other publications. Presently, Constance Young lives in New York City, where she and a group of people are attempting to establish a shelter for stray cats and dogs.